Maroua Garma
Emna Doudech
Adel Bouguezzi

New prospects for autologous grafting in oral surgery

Maroua Garma
Emna Doudech
Adel Bouguezzi

New prospects for autologous grafting in oral surgery

ScienciaScripts

Imprint

Any brand names and product names mentioned in this book are subject to trademark, brand or patent protection and are trademarks or registered trademarks of their respective holders. The use of brand names, product names, common names, trade names, product descriptions etc. even without a particular marking in this work is in no way to be construed to mean that such names may be regarded as unrestricted in respect of trademark and brand protection legislation and could thus be used by anyone.

Cover image: www.ingimage.com

This book is a translation from the original published under ISBN 978-620-6-72584-8.

Publisher:
Sciencia Scripts
is a trademark of
Dodo Books Indian Ocean Ltd. and OmniScriptum S.R.L publishing group

120 High Road, East Finchley, London, N2 9ED, United Kingdom
Str. Armeneasca 28/1, office 1, Chisinau MD-2012, Republic of Moldova, Europe
Printed at: see last page
ISBN: 978-620-8-20782-3

CONTENTS

INTRODUCTION

The last years, we have witnessed à a boomdazzling implantology, which has made dental implants the first choice for replacing missing teeth. This is due to the growing aesthetic and functional demands of patients, who are increasingly tolerant of dental implants. removable solutions less and less.However, these restorations are only possible when the quality and quantity of the bone and gum are satisfactory. In fact, bone and gum defects can represent an obstacle to this procedure.A multitude of strategies, materials and surgical techniques have been developed to overcome these substance deficiencies. Various surgical procedures have been proposed to increase unfavourable bone volume, such as autogenous bone grafts, guided bone regeneration and alveolar distraction osteogenesis(1,2). However, autogenous bone grafts are considered the "gold standard".Another dental tissue, dentin, has recently been studied in all its forms as a new alternative for use as a bone substitute. Numerous reconstructive and regenerative periodontal plastic surgery techniques such as pedicle grafts, free gingival autografts, connective tissue grafts and guided tissue regeneration have also been adopted to treat gingival defects(3). This book is divided into two parts, one devoted to the presentation of two clinical cases illustrating two types of autogenous graft (bone and gingival). The second part will be devoted to a discussion of the different autogenous grafting techniques in terms of interest, indications, limitations, risks and results, as well as innovative procedures.

1ER CASES CLINICAL

A 25-year-old patient consulted the department for functional and aesthetic reasons. He complained of tooth mobility and prosthetic failure in the crowned 21. Questioning revealed that the patient had suffered a previous trauma following a road accident 5 years previously.
The patient is in good health and has no medical or family history that might indicate a need for oral surgery.
On clinical examination, 21 is crowned, has a greyish border at the collar and is mobile degree 2, and 11 is dyschromic with a negative vitality test (fig.1).

Figure 1: Endo buccal examination

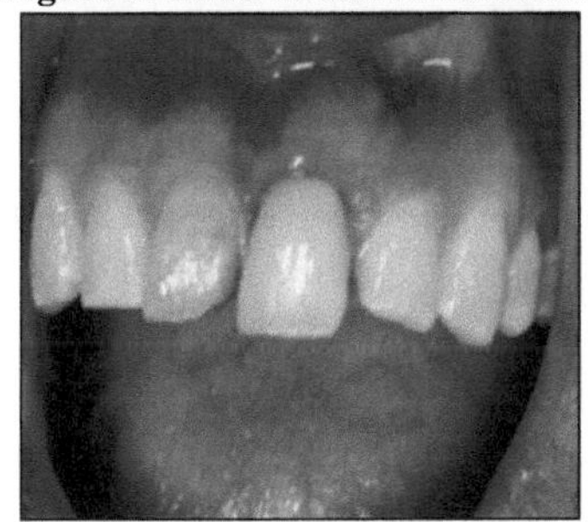

Radiological examination showed a crown with an ill-fitting post on 21, the tooth was treated endodontically and two periapical images related to 11 and 21. Oblique sagittal cone beam sections showed a collapse of the buccal cortex opposite the upper central incisors. (Fig.2)

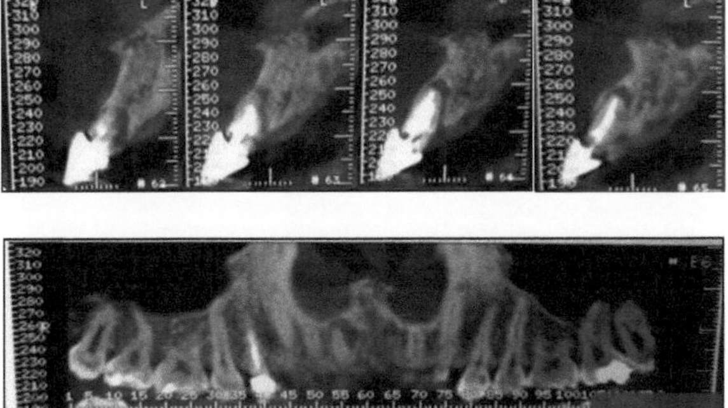

Figure 2: X-ray examination: oblique sagittal sections and curvilinear panoramic reconstruction

Following this examination, a treatment plan was drawn up involving endodontic treatment of tooth 11, extraction of tooth 21 and a pre-implant autogenous bone graft with chin harvesting.

The first session consisted of periodontal cleaning and endodontic treatment of 11, followed by a second session for surgery.

Preparation of the recipient site :

Firstly, the atraumatic extraction of the 21, which was deemed irrecoverable, and the curettage of the two peri-apical lesions were carried out. Vertical bone resorption and insufficient residual vestibulopalatal bone thickness necessitated a pre-implant autogenous bone graft. (Fig.3)

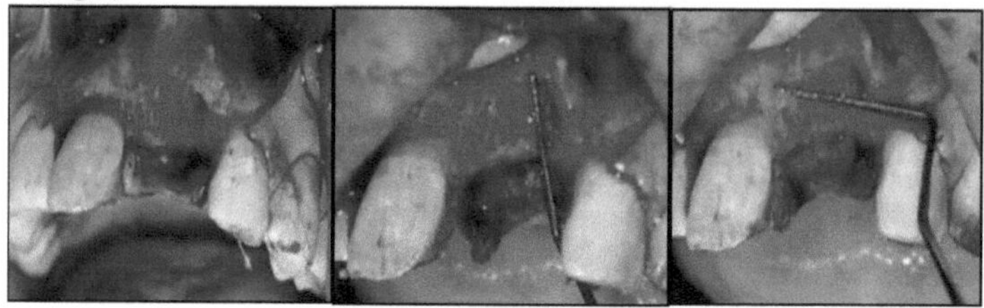

Figure 3: Post-extraction clinical aspect and detached flap: Resorption of the alveolar ridge

Preparation of the donor site :

The choice of a chin harvest was discussed with the patient. A full-thickness para-marginal flap from canine to canine was debonded, a rectangular chin harvest was performed by piezosurgery, then the flap was placed in its initial position and secured with a 3-0 Vicryl absorbable suture (Fig.4).

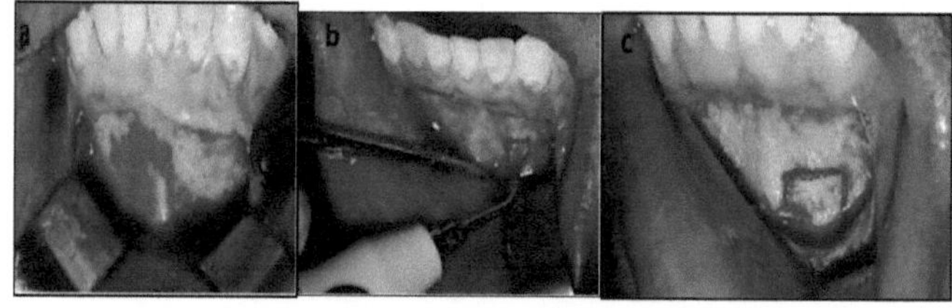

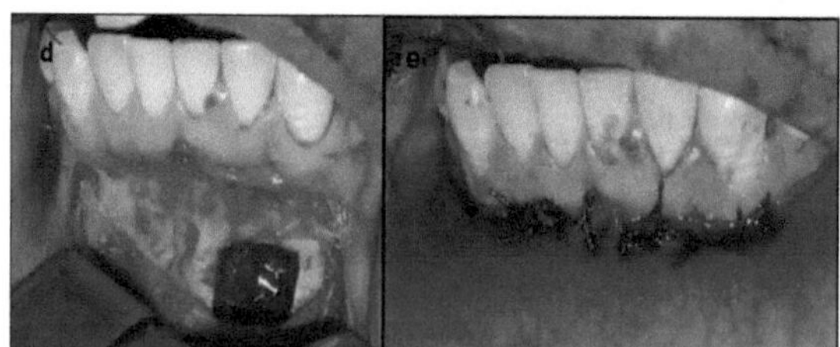

Figure 4: Chin harvesting using piezosurgery

a : Removal of a full-thickness flap,c, d : Preparation of the chin graft e : Sutures

After the edges and angles had been smoothed using the piezosurgery insert, the graft adapted to the recipient site was fixed to the broken vestibular wall at the level of the extracted 21 using an osteosynthesis screw. Bone particles recovered from the preparation of the graft and mixed with physiological saline were added all around the graft to ensure a homogenous transition from the alveolar ridge to the graft. The recipient site was then covered by the repositioned flap and sutured, with a view to a subsequent implant once the graft was well integrated (Fig.5).

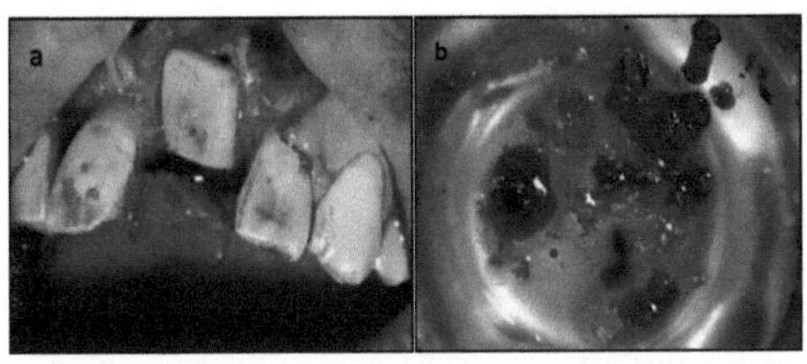

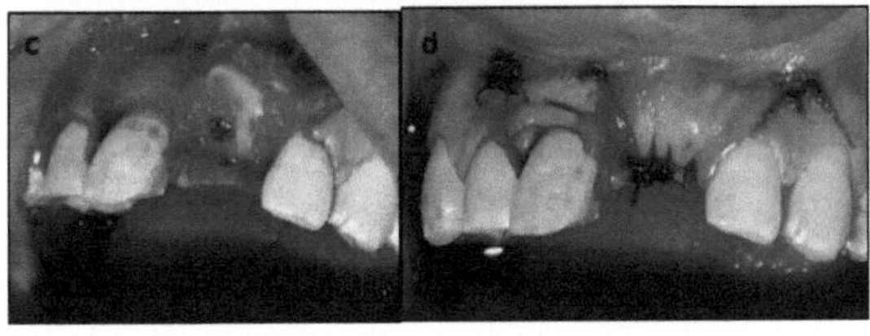

Figure 5: Placing the graft
a : Adaptation of the graft to the recipient site: Recovered bone particlesc :Fixation of the bone block and placement of the particulate bone : Suturing of the flap

2EME CASES CLINICAL

A 58-year-old patient in good general condition was referred to the partial denture department of the University Hospital Clinic of Dental Medicine in Monastir for the removal of a fibrous hyperplasia at the base of the mandibular vestibule and a deepening of the vestibular region for possible total prosthetic rehabilitation stabilised on implants.
The patient was edentulous and had a removable total prosthesis. Exo-oral examination showed a reduction in the vertical dimension of the occlusion. The endo-buccal examination revealed a lesion in the mandible with a pseudo-bite appearance.
hyperplastic tumour in the shape of a "book leaf" in the anterior region of the vestibular fundus. The lesion was covered by non-inflammatory mucosa, was soft to palpation and non-haemorrhagic. The bearing surfaces were very resorbed in the mandible, with a short keratinised mucosa. Examination of the palate revealed an erythema that contrasted sharply with the normal paleness of the mucosa, bordered by the posterior edge of the maxillary prosthesis. This lesion is consistent with subprosthetic candidiasis.

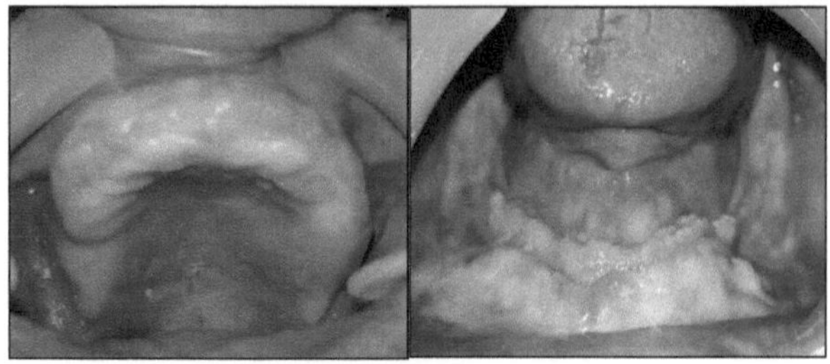

Figure 6: Endo-buccal examination

Analysis of the maxillary prosthesis showed poor maintenance of the prosthesis, associated with a fracture of the repaired maxillary prosthesis.

Following this examination, a surgical-prosthetic treatment plan was proposed to the patient. Firstly, motivation for prosthetic and mucosal hygiene with prescription of a mouthwash composed formed of an antifungal (Fungizone), a 14 ‰ bicarbonate solution and a Chlorhexidine-based antiseptic (Eludril) to be applied 3 to 4 times a day for 21 days was made. This was followed by sessions to monitor the candidiasis under the prosthesis. After 3 weeks from the first consultation, excision of the lesion associated with vestibular deepening was carried out: a local anaesthetic (Mepivacaine 2% with Adrenalin 1: 80,000) was administered to the vestibular mucosa and lip mucosa from the right premolar sector to the left premolar side, followed by a partial-thickness incision, following the limits of the fibrous hyperplasia, which was excised over a width of approximately 10 to 12 mm, extending from the right mandibular 2nd premolar to the contralateral side, thus exposing the underlying connective tissue.

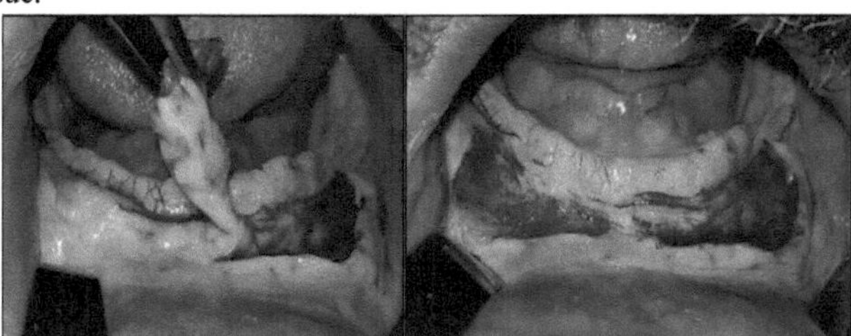

Figure 7: Fissure epulis removal

The lower margin of the incision was sutured in its new position with interrupted periosteal sutures, first at the midline and then at other points along the incision, using 3-0 Vicryl non-absorbable suture.

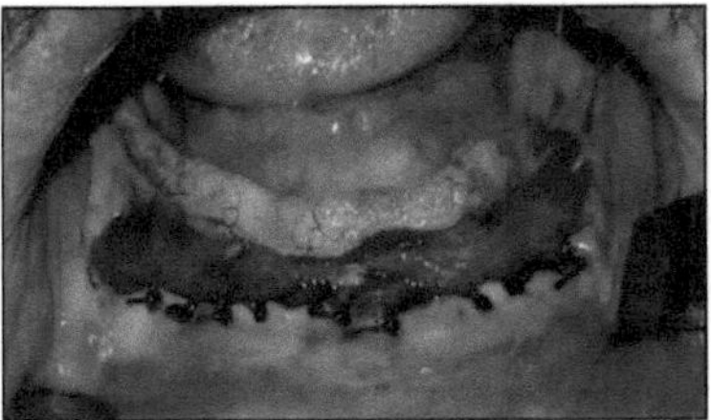

Figure 8: Interrupted periosteal sutures

The epithelial-connective graft was harvested from the palatal mucosa opposite the premolar region at a distance from the top of the ridge, then dissected in partial thickness in order to preserve a layer of connective tissue on the bony surface of the donor site (Fig. 9), and the adipose tissue on its inner surface was then removed (Fig. 10 and Fig. 11).

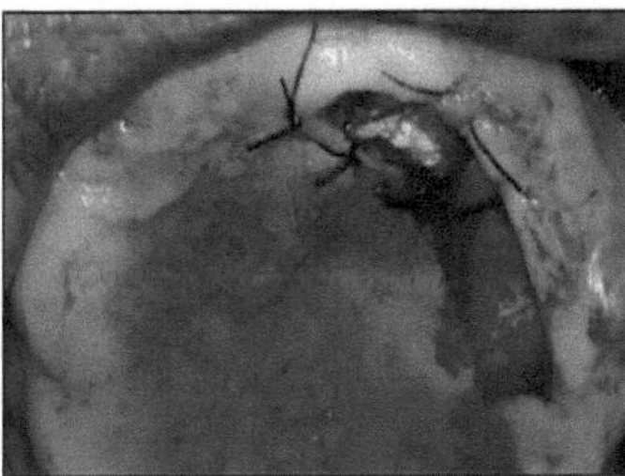

Figure 9: Palatal sampling site

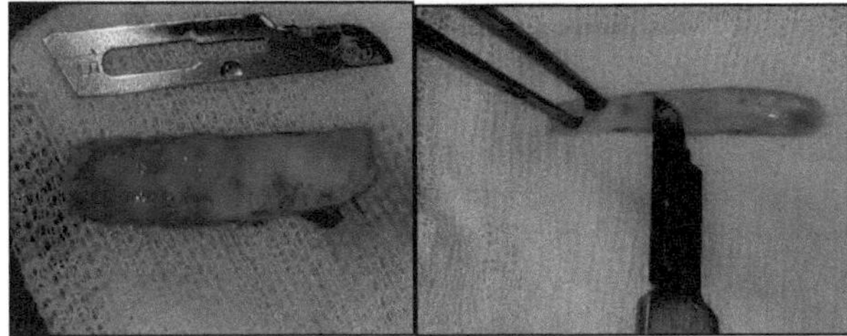

Figure 10: Excised palatal graft

Figure 11: Removal of adipose tissue from the inside of the graft

The graft was then immobilised using simple stitches (at each upper angle), then plated using vertical mattress sutures with periosteal anchoring, to ensure immobilisation in the event of labial traction (Fig. 12).

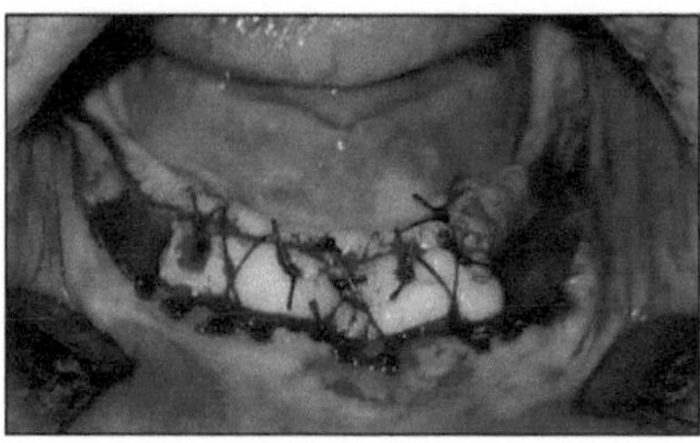

Figure 12: Sutured graft on the recipient site prepared by vestibuloplasty

No periodontal dressing was applied. Post-operative instructions included a soft diet, limited facial movement for 14 days and no brushing around the surgical site for 3 days after surgery, as well as an ice bladder over the lower lip. The patient must rinse gently with a 0.2% Chlorhexidine mouthwash twice a day for 2 weeks. Amoxicillin 2g and ibuprofen 400 mg were prescribed for 5 days. The old total prosthesis was relined using a "Kerr Fit" tissue conditioning material (fig. 13).

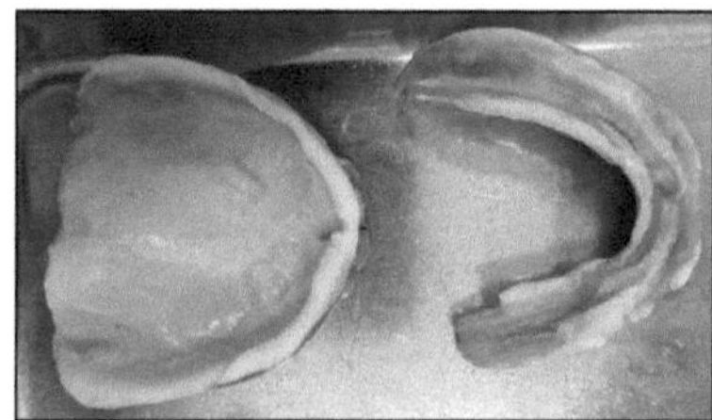

Figure 13: Relining the total prosthesis with the Kerr fit

Favourable post-operative healing was observed two weeks later when the sutures were removed and the patient reported discomfort, particularly at the donor site. Two months later, the definitive total prosthesis was delivered to the patient and perfect integration of the prosthetic volume was noted, as well as retention and stability.that resulted. The vestibuloplasty resulted in a complete mandibular prosthesis that was well extended, stable and retentive. (fig. 14).

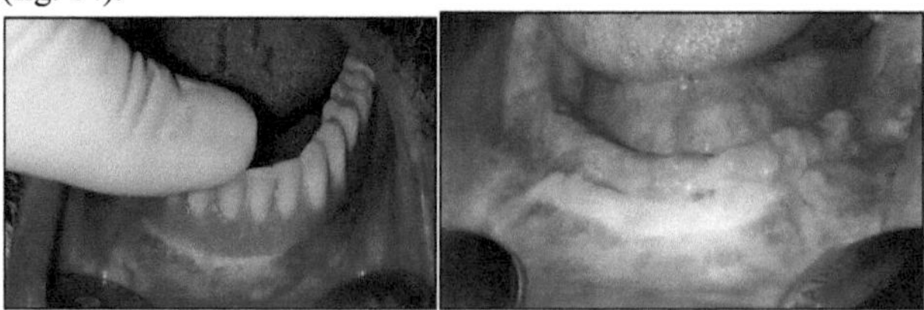

Figure 14: Post-operative status after 2 months

DISCUSSION

I. AUTOGENOUS BONE GRAFT

Bone grafts are procedures for transferring bone tissue of any quality to a recipient bone site, with the aim of increasing bone volume when it is insufficient. This increase provides greater stability and longevity for implant and prosthetic results.

It is an autograft if the graft comes from the recipient himself, which guarantees that it does not provoke any immune reaction and poses no risk of disease transmission.

Autologous bone grafts are considered the "gold standard" for the rehabilitation of atrophic areas, with good reliability and predictability for subsequent implant placement, regardless of the donor area(3).

However, despite a significant number of publications reporting favourable results with these different surgical procedures, considerable controversy remains regarding the choice of the most reliable and appropriate technique, which confers on the bone properties similar to those of the recipient site; this is often due to the lack of comparative studies(1).

1. Interest

1.1. Benefits

Regardless of the site from which it is taken, intra- or extra-oral, G.O.A. remains the procedure of choice, the "gold standard" in bone reconstruction. It has the best immunological, histological and physiological qualities.Autogenous bone has cortical mechanical properties and cancellous bone osteogenic properties that no allograft, xenograft or alloplastic material has been able to achieve.

One of the main advantages of G.O.A. is structural support; bone grafts vary in their ability to bear mechanical load. Cortical grafts can withstand reasonable mechanical loads, whereas cancellous grafts can only resist compression, and even then only to a limited extent. These mechanical properties vary widely depending on the donor site(4,5).

G.O.A. is osteogenic in that it contains cellular elements and growth factors, and is capable of inducing angiogenesis and the growth of mesenchymal stem cells necessary for the formation of new bone(4).Osteoinduction, which refers to the recruitment, proliferation and differentiation of mesenchymal stem cells using growth factors such as bone morphogenetic proteins, is an important property of G.O.A.(4).Through its microscopic matrix, the G.O.A. provides the scaffolding for the cell population essential for bone formation, thus ensuring osteoconduction(4,5). G.O.A. also offers other advantages such as histocompatibility, no risk of disease transmission and less resorption than allografts and xenografts (4)(6).

1.2. Disadvantages

Its limited supply of bone volume, the potential for morbidity and superinfection of the donor site and adjacent structures and the prolonged treatment time are the main hazards of G.O.A.(4,7)(8).

2. Technique

2.1. sampling

A variety of anatomical donor sites may be suitable for harvesting autogenous bone grafts, including the iliac bone, clavicle, ribs, tibia, fibula, coronoid process, zygomatic girdle, maxillary tubercle, mandibular ramus and chin region(8).

2.1.1. Extra- oral sites

2.1.1.1. Fibula (9,10)

It is a versatile free flap that can be used as a bone or osteocutaneous free flap.
This type of graft provides a large calibre of good quality bone capable of being shaped, but requires a long healing period and risks causing complications concerning the mobility of the hallux (9).

2.1.1.2. Bone iliac

The iliac crest is very often used; this site is particularly suitable for reconstruction of the mandible because of the natural contour of the bone, and its crook makes it available for endosseous implants. This iliac crest has a large amount of accessible bone with an appropriate proportion of cortical bone to cancellous bone, but can lead to donor site morbidities including haematoma, numbness in the hip region and hernia formation (9,11). It is more commonly used in the treatment of cancer or trauma requiring large quantities of bone (12)

2.1.1.3. Clavicle

Clavicular bone graft harvesting can be uni-cortical or bi-cortical. The uni-cortical clavicular bone graft has a very good benefit/risk ratio. (13) Its location in the same operating field, making it easier for the patient to settle in, its membranous origin, ensuring less resorption, and the virtual absence of pain and morbidity, add significant value to the harvest. clavicular bone.However, the larger the sample size, the greater the risk of fracture, even if the sample is taken in a single-cortical thickness. Three-dimensional facial reconstruction using clavicular bone is also a difficulty in obtaining the desired shape. There is a general consensus that computer-assisted virtual planning gives more predictable results and is therefore becoming indispensable in reconstructive surgery(11,13).

2.1.1.4. Comparison of different extra- bone grafts

Analysis of bone dimensions using conventional radiographs after fibular and iliac crest grafting showed good vertical maintenance, with reported bone resorption ranging from 0 to 12% in the iliac graft and from 2 to 20% in the fibular graft over a postoperative period of 17 to 47 months(14).The authors (Wilkman et al (15)) observed a continuous decrease in bone volume over time, particularly in free scapular and iliac crest grafts, which continued for several years. The fibular graft showed less loss of bone volume. This stability and reliability of bone volume could be due to the higher cortical bone ratio compared with other commonly used bones. In addition, the fibular graft showed the possibility of appositive bone formation, which led to an increase in bone volume over time. No significant influence of age or adjuvant radiotherapy on graft stability was found. (14) Chen et al(16) describe the superiority of the iliac graft over the fibular graft in terms of postoperative infections, healing rates and pseudarthrosis/union rates.

2.1.2. Intra- oral sites

Intraoral donor sites include the ramus, symphysis, maxillary tuberosity and zygomatic. The ramus and symphysis are considered the most common donor sites for autogenous augmentation (2). These sites offer the advantage of being close to the recipient sites, the absence of skin scars, the possibility of being performed under local anaesthetic and on an outpatient basis, so less stress for the patient, and practical surgical accessibility(8). As a result, intraoral donor sites are generally preferred by surgeons for bone transplantation. The choice of an intraoral donor site generally depends on the volume of replacement bone required and the anatomical situation of the patient(6).

2.1.2.1. The chin region

The chin region is the most commonly used donor site for intraoral autogenous bone grafts.

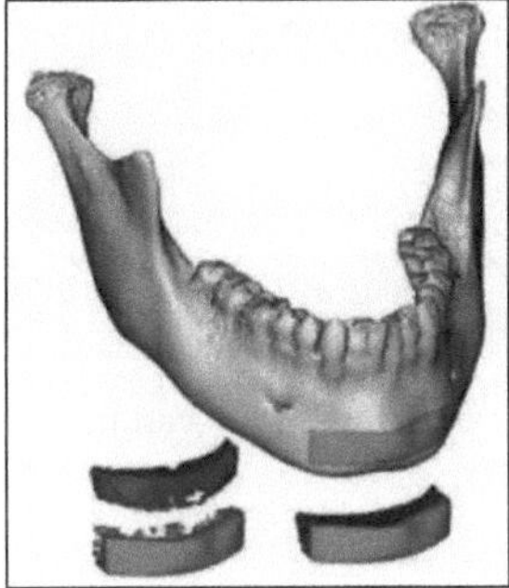

Figure 15: Three-dimensional imagethe volume of symphyseal graft possible Green: the volume of the cortical graftIn red: the volume of the cancellous graft(17).

➤ **Advantages :**

The chin symphysis provides the largest amount of graft material compared to other intra-oral donor sites for alveolar ridge reconstruction.Symphyseal bone is of membranous origin, so it is more resistant to resorption than grafts from endochondral bone and can easily tolerate orthodontic movement of the teeth. The cortical bone taken from this site contains an increased quantity of promoter proteins, and rapid revascularisation of the bone graft is also possible. This donor site is also characterised by its ease of harvesting and the absence of a skin incision. (8)(17,18)

➤ **Disadvantages:**

Harvesting a large quantity of bone carries the risk of altering the contour of the mandible, which could have adverse aesthetic repercussions. In fact, according to research carried out by various studies, there is a residual defect in the mandibular symphysis in all patients undergoing graft removal. The likelihood of residual bone defects is reduced by harvesting a monocortical bone graft.A moderate bone volume of 2.3 ml is estimated for mandibular bone blocks; this quantity is not sufficient for large defects, particularly bilateral clefts(18)(17).

➢ **Postoperative complications** :

Aggravations may be encountered, such as sensory disorders, obliteration and necrosis of the pulp, damage to the bone and bone marrow or even health problems(18).

2.1.2.2. Ramus mandibular

The sampling ramic interests the segment lateral-distal segment of the mandibular body and the anteroinferior segment of the ramus.

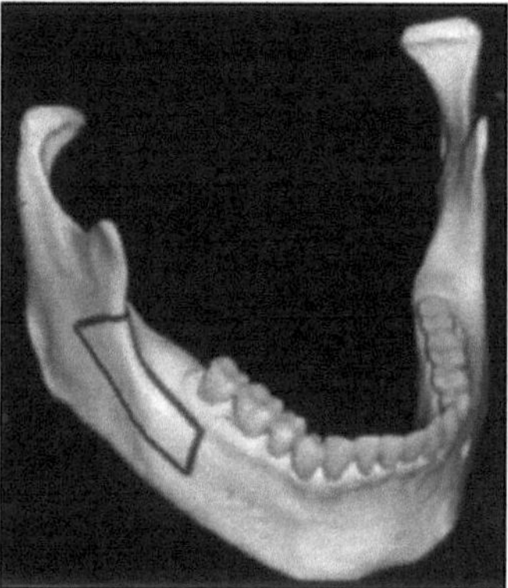

Figure 16: Three-dimensional image the volume of root graft possible (19)

➢ **Advantages** :

A relatively large volume can be successfully removed from the ramus with a low complication rate if the surgical protocol is followed. Despite the fact that a large part of the external oblique line is eliminated, there are virtually no aesthetic or functional consequences. It also has no effect on adjacent teeth(20).
The autogenous bone graft from the mandibular ramus is characterised by dense cortical bone with less cancellous bone, compared with the quality of the bone from the chin graft. (8)

➢ **Disadvantages:**

The surgical approach is relatively more complex than for other sites, and the size of the sample is limited to a rectangular block measuring 30x10x4mm. The morbidity of the donor site is a factor to be taken into account when choosing the mandibular ramus as a source of bone graft,

➢ **Postoperative complications** :

Although postoperative complications have been reported, they are not frequent. Stiffness, limited mobilisation of the vestibule, and altered and decreased sensitivity in adjacent innervated areas can be avoided when appropriate surgical execution is performed. Recovery is influenced by the patient's age and direct surgical injury(21).

2.1.2.3. Palais

The palate offers a number of possible harvesting sites, the retro-incisor region can be considered for small to medium-sized bone reconstruction and the premolar region appears to offer sufficient bone at safe distances from the maxillary sinus and premolar apexes.

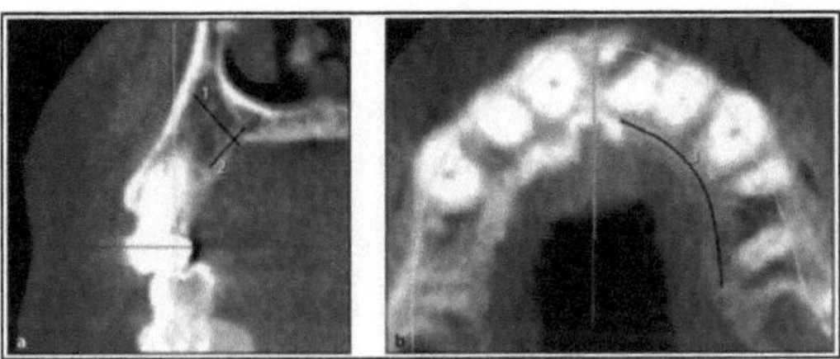

**Figure 17: Horizontal and axial sections of possible palatal graft volume
1 : Maximum width2 : Maximum height3 : maximum length (22)**

> **Benefits**

The benefit/risk ratio is favourable for this type of harvesting, as the donor and recipient sites can be integrated into the same surgical field, which can limit the post-operative course. It also offers an easily accessible harvesting zone and a sufficient quantity of bone to treat a bone defect in a single implant or two implants, with the possibility of bilateral harvesting to increase the volume of autogenous bone available, while limiting the safety distances with respect to neighbouring anatomical structures (22)(23).

> **Disadvantages**

The amount of bone that can be harvested from the palate is low, due to the presence of the incisal canal, the nasal floor, the maxillary sinus and the roots of the maxillary teeth. These bone volume values may be influenced by external factors, such as the wearing of braces in the past or a history of surgery in these areas. (22)(23)

> **Post-operative complications :**

Studies of post-operative follow-up show that patients do not feel any discomfort at the donor site and that pain is relatively low. In vivo studies show a very low failure rate(23).

2.1.2.4. Maxillary tuberosity

Grafts from the maxillary tuberosity are more accessible and offer better post-operative results than mandibular intra-oral sites. The maxillary tuberosity has the lowest values in terms of bone density as well as a very thin cortex, which can lead to a high risk of resorption, and allows small quantities of grafts to be used(22).This location presents the risk of intruding into the sinus and the risk of invading the Bichat's ball(23).

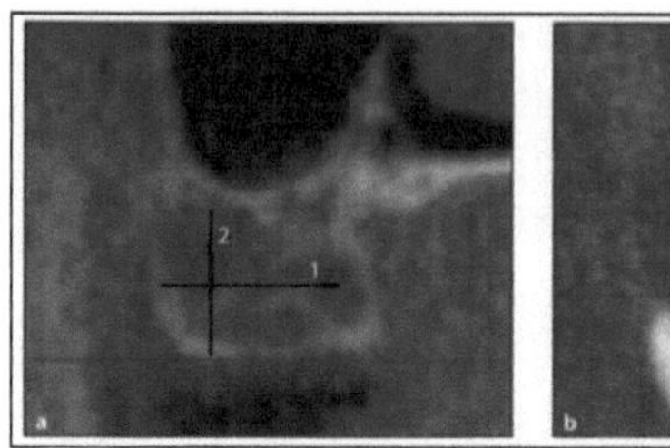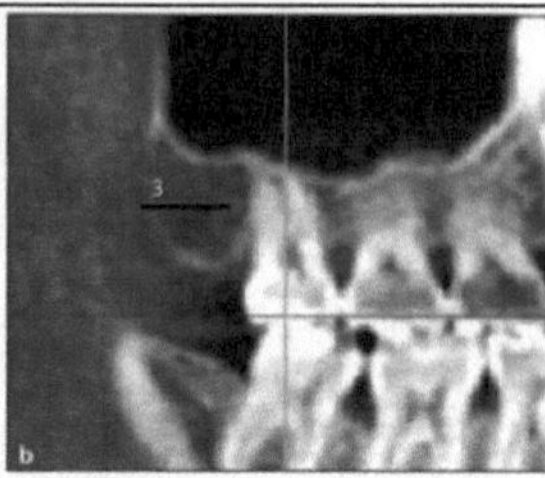

Figure 18: Coronal oblique section and panoramic reconstruction of possible tuberosity graft 1 : Maximum width 2 : Maximum height 3 : maximum length (22)

2.1.2.5. Comparison of different intra- oral grafts

➤ **Bone quality :**

Studies have shown that early horizontal resorption (4 months after bone grafting) of the ramus graft was significantly lower than that of the chin graft. In addition, the residual thickness of the bone plate grafted from the ramus was significantly greater than that from the chin.

To investigate why branch grafting had better graft stability, the following factors known to affect autogenous bone graft resorption were analysed:

(1) The embryonic origin of the graft (membranous bone grafts have minimal resorption compared to endochondral bone),

(2) Ratio of cortical bone to cancellous bone,

(3) The adaptation of bone grafts to recipient sites is essential for its incorporation, which is a process in which bone tissue from the recipient site grows into the bone graft and then forms haversian systems. Bone tissue migrates smoothly into the bone graft only if the bone graft is in close contact with the recipient site, which is also beneficial for revascularisation of the graft by preventing micromovements.

The ramus and symphysis are both membranous bone, but the vast majority of grafts in the ramus are cortical bone and those in the symphysis are cortico-cancellous bone.

Cortical bone has better mechanical strength to maintain the volume of the graft and transfer the biting forces after loading(2).

➤ **Complications :**

There appears to be a trend towards a higher pain score, and more prolonged pain and increased need for analgesics after autogenous bone graft harvesting in the chin region compared with the mandibular ramus according to questionnaire and VAS, although pain during chewing was significantly greater after harvesting in the mandibular ramus.(8)

No difference in infections after autogenous bone graft harvesting in the chin or ramus region has been reported in several studies. No differences in mucosal dehiscence following autogenous bone graft harvesting in the chin or mandibular ramus region were reported.

Statistical research found that altered sensation of the lower incisors was reported by 29% of patients after autogenous bone graft harvesting from the chin region, whereas no alteration in sensation of adjacent teeth was reported after harvesting from the mandibular ramus(8).

However, the selection of a specific intraoral donor site for the harvesting of an autogenous bone graft is based on various aspects including the surgeon's preference, the quantity and quality of bone required, access to the donor site, and potential surgical complications.

2.2. Comparison between types of bone grafts autogenous

The procedure chosen for bone augmentation should be the simplest and least invasive, with the lowest risk of complications in the shortest time. The surgeon and patient must weigh up the advantages and disadvantages of the procedures to be selected. (3)

2.2.1. Comparison between cancellous autograft and cortical autograft

Bone grafts, whether autograft or allograft, are described as cortical or cancellous, depending on the type of bone harvested. Bone autografts can be classified into two categories: non-vascularised and vascularised.

	Cancellous autograft	Cortical autograft
Benefits	+ Three-dimensional porous scaffolding :	+ Osteoconductor
	highly osteo-conductive	+ Better structural support
	+ Osteocytes and stem cells as well as	
	than spinal cord cells:	
	osteogenic	
	+ Growth factors: osteoinductive	
Disadvantages	- Initial poor structural support	- Less biological activity
	improves as the bone forms.	than cancellous grafts:
		less surface area and fewer
		cellular matrix than bone
		spongy
		- More time for
		revascularisation
Website of	the iliac crest, the posterior iliac spine-	Ramus
sampling	the femur, the tibia, the radius or the	Chin region
	the maxillary tuberosity.	

2.2.2. Comparison between en bloc autograft and particulate

An autogenous bone block has better mechanical resistance than particulate bone, and therefore demonstrates superiority in the repair of severe horizontal bone defects with a flat bone arch morphology and vertical defects.
Autogenous bone block grafting is considered the preferred modality for repairing Terheyden 2/4 and 3/4 bone defects. However, a bone block graft presents the problem of poor adaptation to the recipient bed, which can lead to longer healing times and a lower success rate(2).

2.3. Different techniques

The selection of the ideal grafting technique is a highly debatable multifactorial subject depending mainly on each clinical situation such as the dimensions of the remaining available bone, the proximity of vital structures, the quality of the soft tissues, the systemic state of the patient and the preferences and skills of the operator(24).

2.3.1. Free grafts vascularised

The vascularised fibula osteocutaneous flap has been well described in the literature as the first choice reconstructive option for maxillectomy defects. It is a flap capable of providing immediate reconstruction with the possibility of immediate dental implants. They allow the reconstruction of composite defects in both soft tissue and bone(9).
Microvascular bone reconstruction plays an important role in restoring the oro-mandibular unit and optimises aesthetic and functional results, particularly in patients without adjuvant radiotherapy(14).
Mandibular reconstruction remains a major morphological and functional challenge. The currently accepted gold standard for reconstruction of large mandibular defects is the use of free autologous bone flaps(14).

> **Computer-assisted surgery :**

Computer Assisted Surgery (CAS), which is frequently used to describe surgery; where planning, rapid prototyping of surgical guide and models, and recently pre-identification of drill holes, nerves and tumour margins can be achieved. Recent advances include preoperative rehabilitation planning beyond bone reconstruction, such as Jaw In A Day(9,25).
Virtual surgical planning has gained significant popularity and widespread use due to improved surgical precision and reduced operative time. Most current maxillofacial CT scanners and cone-beam CT scanners acquire sufficient data to perform this task, although 1 mm sections from the maxillofacial scanner are ideal. Firstly, it allows surgeons to carry out their surgery pre-operatively and plan ahead in their minds, enabling them to visualise possible difficulties and complications. Secondly, with a 'wrap' of the tumour, you can plan the resection margins in the three-dimensional (3D) viewpoint and thus classify the reconstruction according to the defect expected after application of the surgical margin.Thirdly, using mirroring capabilities, advanced tactile models can be created where plates could be pre-formed or PSI could be created with 3D printing. 3D printing options include titanium, PEEK (polyetheretherketone) or PEKK (polyetherketoneketone). Finally,

recent advances with predictive screw holes, endosseous implants and immediate nerve grafts allow faster reconstruction with optimal dental and neural rehabilitation. (9) (25)

Computer-assisted surgery (CAS) for mandibular reconstruction is booming, and there are an increasing number of indications for maxillofacial reconstruction. The use of customised cutting guides for this indication considerably reduces surgical times, improves dental restoration and postoperative appearance, and appears to improve the accuracy of the reconstruction.However, the cost of the procedure remains quite exorbitant for patients. Some authors have developed a "universal" cutting guide for fibular osteotomies to obtain a symphysis angle of 120° and a symphysis length of 25 mm. We believe it is unnecessary to distinguish between male and female mandibular reconstructions. The "universal cutting guide", designed using anatomical means, would broaden the indications for guided mandibular reconstructions, allowing a greater number of patients to benefit from guided reconstructions, without high cost and manufacturing time.(26)

2.3.2. Non vascularised graft

Autogenous bone blocks can act as an osteo-conductive scaffold for vascular and cellular growth, maintaining a constant and adequate volume for constant remodelling and adequate mineralisation. Block grafts also demonstrate better formation of vital and mineralised bone with lamellar organisation at the graft sites compared with other grafts(27).

Free bone grafts must be small to survive as there is no intrinsic blood supply. These grafts are thought to be at greater risk of resorption over time due to their dependence on adjacent vascularisation(28).

Another consideration when using non-vascularised bone grafts is the potential need for adjuvant radiation. Radiation can increase the risk of non-union, resorption and material extrusion, so the histology of the tumour and the potential need for adjuvant treatment must be taken into account when choosing the reconstruction.(28)

2.3.2.1. Graft onlay

This type of graft is used to reconstruct the maxillary or mandibular crest. The aim is to obtain a volume of bone compatible with the functional and aesthetic placement of a dental implant and its prosthesis.It can be transverse to treat horizontal defects or vertical to treat vertical defects. height deficiencies with a lower success rate.

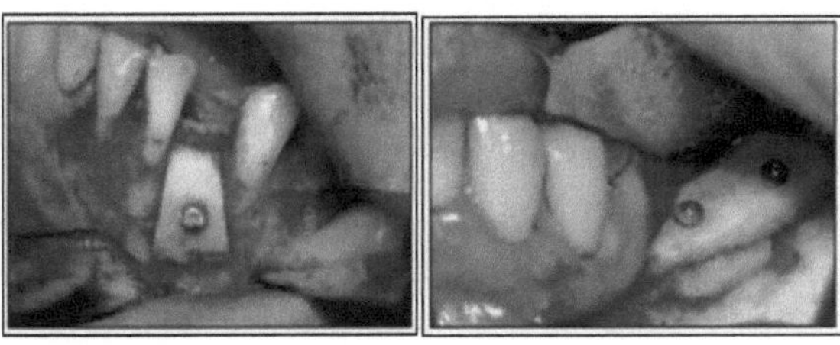

Figure 19 and 20: Horizontal and vertical onlay grafts in trans-veneered blocks

> **Indications:**

The transverse onlay graft is used to re-establish maxillomandibular relationships and alignment compatible with a stable occlusion of the future prosthesis, while the vertical onlay graft is used to correct the relative position of the inferior alveolar nerve, which constitutes the main anatomical limits. This vertical apposition will also be indicated in cases where the prosthetic space is greatly increased, in order to ensure better aesthetic and functional integration of the implant-supported crown(29).

The onlay block autograft technique with immediate implant placement could lead to increased osseointegration with better primary fixation and graft stability at the recipient site, thus improving the success rates of the procedure and minimising the amount of crestal bone loss that occurs mainly after graft placement. This combined procedure also reduces the number of surgeries required for bone reconstruction, thereby reducing patient discomfort following multiple surgeries in the same area(24) (30).

> **Disadvantages :**

Onlay bone grafts stretch and deform the overlying soft tissue envelope, generating recoil forces that act directly on the en bloc graft. This could explain the significant amount of graft resorption found in several studies(24,30).

> **Complications :**

Flap dehiscence and exposure of the graft during healing have been noted in a few patients who have undergone this type of surgery within a short period of time. time ranging from 10 days to 2 months. It was also reported that the exposed part of the en bloc graft showed clinical signs of necrosis three weeks later.

Management of the complication is either daily irrigation with normal saline, or rounding and minimisation of the exposed part of the graft en bloc with re-closure of the flap (24).

2.3.2.2. Interpositional graft: sandwich

Interposition bone grafting can be performed in the mandible and maxilla to compensate for transverse or vertical bone defects. It consists of performing an osteotomy to create a space between two pedicled bone volumes, and interposing bone(29).

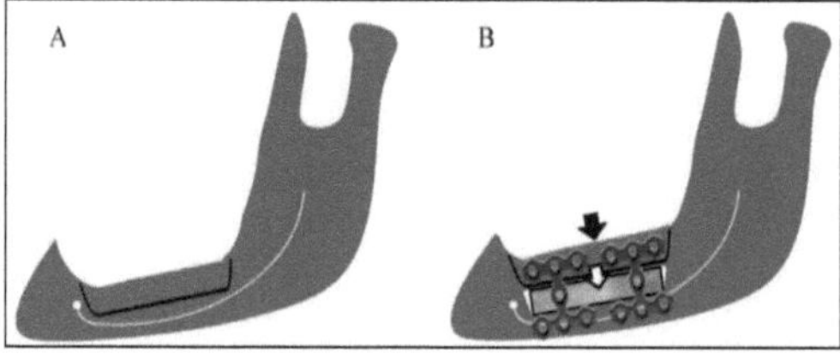

Figure 21: The interpositional grafting technique

A: Trapezoidal osteotomy; B: Elevated segment and cortico-cancellous graft fixed with mini-plates (31)

➢ **Advantages :**

The base and sides of the graft are in intimate contact with the recipient bed. The result is a contact surface between the graft and the host that is more than doubled. This increased contact leads to greater graft-host interaction.
Interpositional grafting converts the single-wall defect into a four-wall defect. Cortellini et al (32) demonstrated that bone filling improved significantly as the number of residual defect walls increased.The graft also remains protected from any harmful stresses that fall on the alveolar ridge. Placing the graft between two pedicled bone layers accelerates angiogenesis in the graft, resulting in increased potential for osteo-inductive and osteo-conductive activity and greater biological activity.
This could be considered superior to onlay block grafting where angiogenesis occurs mainly in one direction and contact between graft and host is also reduced(33).

➢ **Indications:**

Interpositional grafting allows an implant to be placed in thin bone ridges after separating the palatal and vestibular (or lingual) bone cortices, but requires a minimum thickness of 3mm to attempt to split the ridge. This allows a minimum of 1mm of buccal and lingual cortex and 1mm of cancellous bone in between to facilitate splitting and mobilisation of the buccal plate.
The anteroposterior extent of the defect is also an important factor: Longer defects (spaces of three or more teeth) were more difficult to separate due to the inherent rigidity of the mandibular bone. In such cases, dividing the long segment by a vertical cut into two smaller ones facilitated division and mobilisation. (30,33)

➢ **Operating protocol :**

Vertical corticotomies should be relatively parallel or slightly convergent towards the crest. Care must be taken not to encroach on adjacent roots.
The three cuts must extend into the cancellous bone and must be connected together to allow mobilisation of the buccal segment(33).
Care must be taken not to strip the periosteum crestally and palatally to avoid resorption of the crestal bone after the grafting procedures(24).
Interpositional fixation of bone grafts was another point of debate. Some studies used mini-plates to stabilise the mobilised segment. Another study reported that it is not necessary to fix the mobilised segment. Some authors advocate fixation of the osteotomised segment with dental implants immediately to eliminate any micromovement in the graft-native bone interphase, which could increase its resorption(24).

2.3.2.3. Bone ring graft

The bone ring technique allows three-dimensional reconstruction of alveolar bone defects in the aesthetic zone using ring-shaped autogenous bone grafts and simultaneous placement of dental implants in a one-stage procedure.This technique provides three-dimensional augmentation with simultaneous implant placement in a one-stage procedure. In addition, the treatment period required for this technique is shorter than that for other grafting techniques(6).

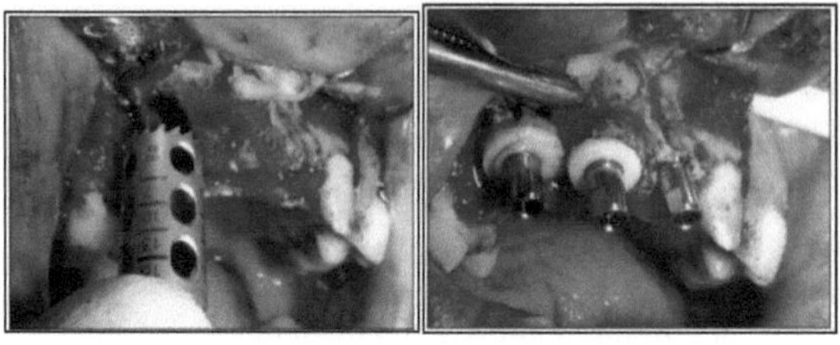

Figure 22: Bone ring grafting

A: Trepan burr measuring the defective socket + implant osteotomy

B: Final position of grafts and implants (6)

➤ **Sampling sites :**

The mandibular symphysis, ramus and maxillary tubercle region are suitable as local / intra-oral donor sites for cortico-cancellous bone.

The quality (density) of the newly formed bone is directly dependent on the qualities of the graft, including the presence of growth factors, favourable modelling and remodelling characteristics, reduction of micro-motion of the graft and its osteo-conductive properties(27).

➤ **Advantages ;**

Bone ring grafting ensures horizontal and vertical bone gain with minimal marginal bone loss while retaining viable osteoblasts and no immunological response. The grafted bone is more rigid and resistant than particulate bone grafts(27).

➤ **Operating protocol :**

The trapezoidal incision at the donor site is followed by a full-thickness detachment. A drill bit was used to remove the bone cylinder with a diameter greater than that of the defect in the recipient site. After making the bone annular discs, an implant osteotomy was made in the centre of the annular graft under copious irrigation, taking care not to perforate the lingual side- A lifting ring was then used to harvest the ring block graft.

The defective area was first prepared using the trepan burr to adapt the bone ring graft to the recipient area. Once the graft had been positioned, the planned implant was inserted through the bone ring, then fixed and immobilised. The augmented area was then covered with a barrier membrane for additional protection against the bone resorption process(6).

2.3.3. Tenting cortical

The combination of 3D reconstruction using a bone block filled with particulate bone is a simple and effective treatment that offers good short-term results, minimal complications and good stability over time(3). Tenting has been recommended for the reconstruction of maxillofacial defects. Various techniques have been reported, the first being the "Tent-pole. The other two modifications, the autogenous cortical tent and the screw tent, are generally used for small oral anomalies. Studies have shown that they can all be used to effectively augment bone(34).

➢ **Principle :**

This technique, based on the principles of guided bone regeneration, involves lifting the periosteum like a tent to allow osteoblasts to migrate into the space to start osteogenesis. The space created is then filled with osteoconductive or osteoinductive materials, or in some cases both.
The migration of epithelial cells can be prevented by the application of a barrier-type collagen membrane or other component.
The technique is divided into three categories depending on the method used to maintain the periosteum(35).

2.3.3.1. Tenting technique- pole

In this procedure, dental implants are used to create a space between the periosteum and the bone and, in most cases, the space is filled with bone grafts.

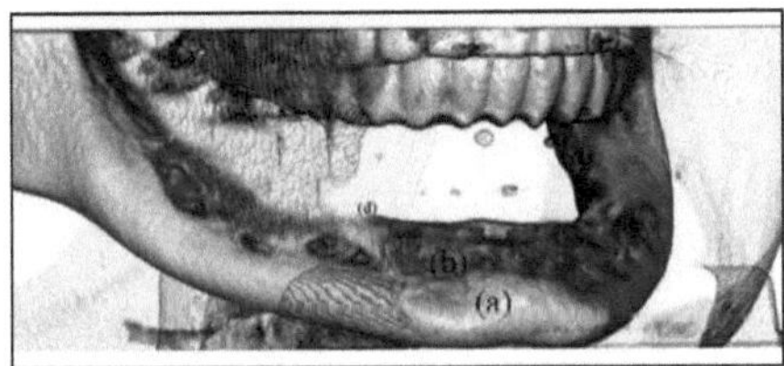

Figure 23: Three-dimensional representation of the "technical tent-pole".

a : basal boneb: iliac bone graftc: dental implant d: periosteum (34)

➢ **Advantages :**

Use of the technique resulted in bone height gains of up to 10 mm. Long-term follow-up (over five years) showed that the augmentation was reliable, with minimal resorption and successful implants (36).
Although more complicated than the other two, the technique can result in a higher vertical height, and may be the only suitable method for reconstructing severely atrophic objects.

➢ **Disadvantage :**

This technique results in incorrect angulation of the implants, in many cases preventing the prostheses from being made. It requires an extra-oral incision (the other two techniques use an intra-oral approach).

➢ **Complications :**

The tent-pole may cause transient or permanent paresthesia of the inferior alveolar nerve and may require a second operation such as vestibuloplasty (35,36).

2.3.3.2. Tent at screws

In this method, titanium screws are used to fill the gap. The space is filled with bone material, and a membrane is used to prevent epithelial cell migration.The face, which is relatively simple and does not involve the harvesting of a bone graft, is associated with low morbidity and can be performed in patients with narrow, atrophic maxillary ridges.

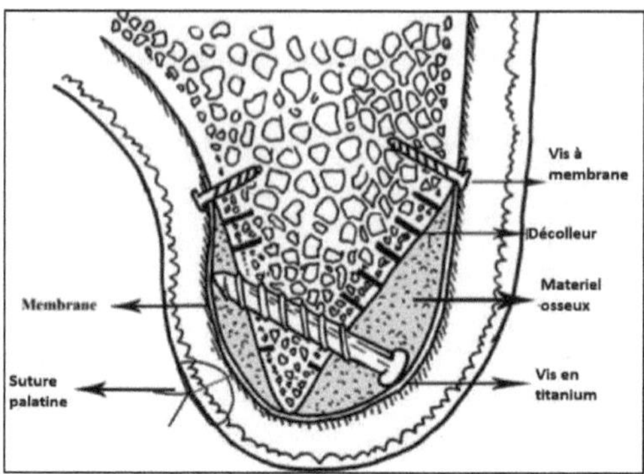

Figure 24: Diagram of the screw tent technique(6)

> **Indications**:

It is particularly indicated for augmentation of atrophic maxillary ridges and partially edentulous short ridges.

> **Complications :**

Dehiscence or infection of the wound and exposure of the screw.

> **Contraindications:**

As bone resorption is relatively high, the technique is not suitable for vertical augmentation, or horizontal augmentation of atrophic ridges (three-dimensional reconstruction), or large defects (34,35).

2.3.3.3. Comparison of the two techniques

Bone height gains were lower than those reported using the tent-pole technique. The technique is best suited to defects in the anterior maxilla, while the tent-pole procedure is best used in the posterior mandible. The tent-pole technique is used to gain bone height, but the screw tent is mainly used for horizontal augmentation.The results of these studies suggest that screw placement may be the best technique for increasing the width of a short-span alveolar ridge prior to implant placement. (3)

2.3.3.4. Autogenic tent cortical

This technique (sometimes called the shell technique) was first described by Le et al(37), who fixed a block of cortical bone with titanium screws a few millimetres from the bone to make the hole, which was filled with bone material. The space between the bone block and the surface of the alveolar crest was filled with autogenous bone (3).

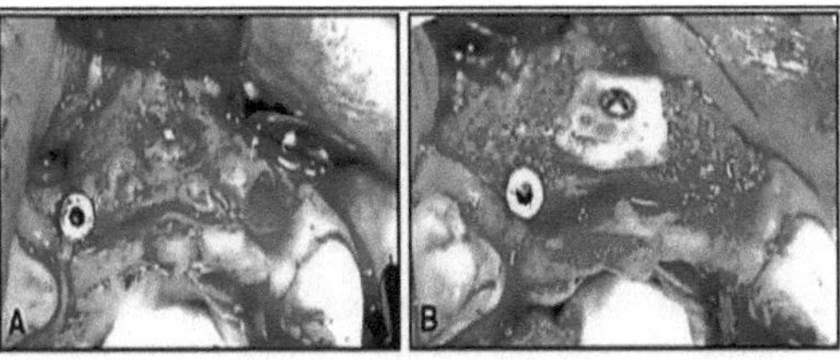

Figure 25: Cortical tenting technique

A: Resorbed alveolar ridgeB: Particulate graft placed around the en bloc graft to "tempt" the periosteum to prevent resorption.

➤ **Advantages :**

The combination of 3D reconstruction using a bone block divided into two thin layers and filled with bone particles is a simple and effective treatment that offers good short-term results, minimal complications and good long-term stability(3).

➤ **Indications:**

Mainly used in the posterior mandible

➤ **Complications :**

The most common complications are wound infection, graft exposure or failure, and bone resorption (34).

2.3.3.5. Khoury and al technique

Khoury et al(38) used a different version of the tenting technique for three-dimensional reconstruction of atrophic mandibular ridges. They divided a cortical bone graft that had been harvested from the lateral ramus of the mandible into two, fixed the two strips in three dimensions and filled the space underneath with bone material.

This technique, which is mainly used for vertical augmentation of the posterior mandible and horizontal augmentation of the anterior maxilla, can increase the ridge by up to 5 mm. The results reported in studies using cortical tenting and screw tenting to widen the anterior maxilla were similar. (34)

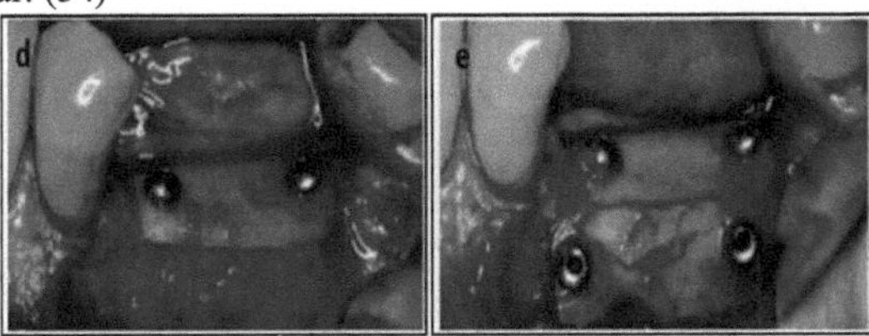

Figure 26: Modified cortical tenting technique

a: atrophic alveolar ridge b: donor site c: bone block divided in twod: occlusal part of the graft stabilised by two screws and space filled with bone particles e: stabilised vestibular part(3)

2.3.4. Technique for removing bone debris

In clinical practice, various harvesting techniques have been used to collect autogenous bone particles during implant surgery, and different techniques can influence osteogenesis and graft resorption(39).
A key to the success of autografting was revealed when researchers showed that "osteogenic cells in the bone itself" contributed directly to new bone formation(40).

2.3.4.1. Bone trap filter technique

The implant bed for insertion of oral implants is usually prepared using high-speed drilling with cold water irrigation. A bone trap filter was used to collect bone particles.
This procedure is considered to be a conservative technique, as it is not necessary to open up a second surgical area.
However, many more micro-organisms were found in the bone particles harvested by this method, resulting in a greater biological risk. Furthermore, in this study, the bone particles obtained were not competitive with the other methods in terms of osteoblast activity and osteogenic potential (39).

2.3.4.2. Bone scraper technique

Cortical bone particles obtained using a bone scraper had a positive effect on bone generation, resulting in a stable bone augmentation effect. These particles also performed well in terms of the biological activity of osteoblasts.
However, the quantity of particles depended on the quality and density of the alveolar bone and an additional flap operation, or even the opening of a second operating zone, is often necessary to expose the scraped area(39).

2.3.4.3. Low-speed drilling

The low-speed drilling system (50 rpm), without additional irrigation, makes it possible to obtain live autogenous bone particles. This method requires no additional operative steps and causes no additional damage to the surrounding bone. The low speed means that no additional heat is generated that could damage the bone, compared with drilling at 900 rpm under irrigation.
Bone particles obtained by low-speed drilling have a high cell content, a high capacity for osteoblasts to proliferate, migrate, differentiate and produce mineralised tissue, high gene transcription and high secretion of proteins linked to osteogenesis.
The quantity of bone particles harvested by low-speed drilling is generally twice the quantity of bone particles harvested by a scraper in a single tooth implantation zone.
Moreover, from a histological point of view, tissue samples taken by low-speed drilling contain more abundant growth factors than those taken by a scraper, and have a high induction capacity conducive to early vascularisation and subsequent osteogenesis of the graft zone, since the former include not only cortical but also cancellous bone (3,39).

3. Complications associated with bone grafts

Younger and Chapman(41) reviewed 243 procedures and documented an overall major complication rate of 8.6%.Complications included infection, prolonged wound drainage, re-operation, pain lasting more than 6 months and sensory loss.Minor complications, described as superficial infection, minor wound problems, temporary sensory loss, and mild or resolving pain occurred in 20.6% of patients.The morbidity of autologous bone harvesting clearly depends on the choice of donor site.Morbidity associated with the use of the iliac crest has been well documented and includes haemorrhage, fractures, neurological injury and significant pain. There may be fewer complications associated with the use of the posterior iliac crest compared to the anterior crest. However, the morbidity of iliac crest grafts appears to be less with smaller grafts.
Pain, swelling, bleeding, infection, dehiscence, dysaesthesia or loss of vitality of the tooth, limited opening of the mouth, changes in the contour of the donor area, and transient or permanent neurosensory disturbances of the inferior alveolar nerve are the complications most frequently reported after intraoral autogenous bone graft harvesting(4) (42).

4. Conclusion

Reporting or comparing the results of any bone grafting technique is complicated by the heterogeneous nature of the studies reported, many of which are simple case series, the various aetiologies of the bone defect, the site of the defect, differences in patient selection, differences in graft harvesting technique, graft preparation or insertion, and the method of bone stabilisation used(4).It is recommended that the patient adhere to a strict pureed diet for a few months after reconstruction to allow adequate healing and union of the bone segments(9).

II.   GINGIVAL GRAFT AUTOGENOUS

A gingival graft is a piece of epithelial and/or connective tissue freed from any blood supply and reimplanted to be integrated by the surrounding native tissue(43).
Since its introduction over 50 years ago, soft tissue grafting has been increasingly used in clinical practice to increase tissue thickness, restore an adequate width of keratinised tissue, correct mucogingival deformities and improve the aesthetics of teeth and dental implant sites(44).The importance of having an adequate width and thickness of keratinised tissue appears to be crucial for both natural teeth and dental implants. In fact, just as teeth lacking keratinised tissue have been shown to be more prone to further loss of attachment, a lack of keratinised mucosa around implants has been shown to impede the patient's oral and dental hygiene, leading to greater soft tissue inflammation, mucosal recession and loss of attachment. In addition, it has been reported that peri-implant soft tissue thickness can also affect marginal bone loss(44,45).

1. Techniques

Various methods of defect correction are possible and the procedure to be chosen depends on local anatomical conditions, the choice of operator and patient comfort(47).

1.1. Gingival graft free

Although the role of keratinised tissue in maintaining peri-implant health is not uniformly accepted, several trials have shown that soft tissue augmentation using free gingival grafting is effective in reducing mucosal inflammation, patient discomfort and facilitating optimal plaque control around implants(44).Patients' growing interest in aesthetics has led to a refinement of the objectives of mucogingival surgery. Free gingival grafting continues to be a reliable and highly predictable procedure for increasing the width of the gingiva. keratinised tissue, stop the progression of gingival recession and thus create an adequate band of keratinised tissue (47)(48).

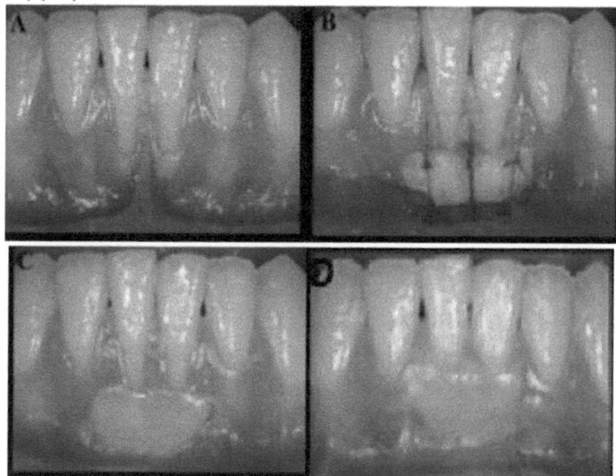

Figure 27: Free gingival graftingin the lower central incisors

(A): Pre-operative condition (B): Direct post-operative condition (C): 5 months post-operatively (D): After 6 months: Complete coverage of defects with keratinised gingiva (44)

1.1.1 Benefits

This technique is simple, with easy tissue handling, allowing several teeth to be treated at the same time. It offers the greatest capacity for increasing the width of the keratinised tissue of all the other types of graft, and eliminates the need for brakes(47) (44).

1.1.2. Disadvantages

The main disadvantage of free gingival grafting is the lack of predictability in terms of aesthetics: poor colour matching with the surrounding tissue, which limits the indication for free gingival grafting to non-aesthetic areas. (48)(47)

It is also limited by the availability of autologous grafting, which may be inadequate when treating several augmentation sites. Palatal harvesting, for example, is influenced by the anatomy of the arch, age, sex, age of the patient and the type of augmentation. population and the variability of the great palatine artery and its branches which make it impossible to draw a definitive conclusion and to provide universal guidelines for "safe" sampling(44,45).

1.1.3. Complications

L.G.A. can have aesthetic complications, such as a massive appearance in the event of poor technique or the risk of having a texture similar to scar tissue.
At the donor site, harvesting may result in prolonged intraoperative and postoperative bleeding or palatal sensory dysfunction (for palatal harvesting). (48)

1.1.4. Indications

One of the major indications for free gingival grafting is to re-establish adequate keratinised tissue and gingival thickness in the presence of muco-gingival defects. It also increases the vestibular depth and width of the keratinised tissue prior to implant reconstruction and root coverage. (44)
Cortellini et al(49) introduce a modification of the conventional approach for its use in root canal coverage: "partially epithelialised graft".The aim is to improve the aesthetic appearance of the "alveolar mucosa" in the anterior inferior zone to compensate for the aesthetic deficiencies that have been reported and to increase the percentage of average root coverage, at the same time facilitating ideal repositioning of the alveolar mucosa(45).

1.1.5. Protocol

Over the last decade, improved techniques and the introduction of the microsurgical approach, consisting of magnification, illumination, micro-instruments and new suture materials, have contributed to greater predictability in root canal procedures(44).
Free gingival grafting can be performed in one or two stages. The technique proposed by Miller(50) is a one-stage procedure also known as the direct approach, while that described by Bernimoulin et al.(51) involves two surgical stages and is known as the indirect approach(47).

1.2. Connective tissue graft

The increasing shift from free gingival grafting to connective tissue grafting represents the transition from traditional mucogingival surgery to periodontal plastic surgery (44).
At present, free gingival grafts lag behind connective tissue grafts, which are generally considered to be the gold standard for managing the height and width of keratinised tissue(47).

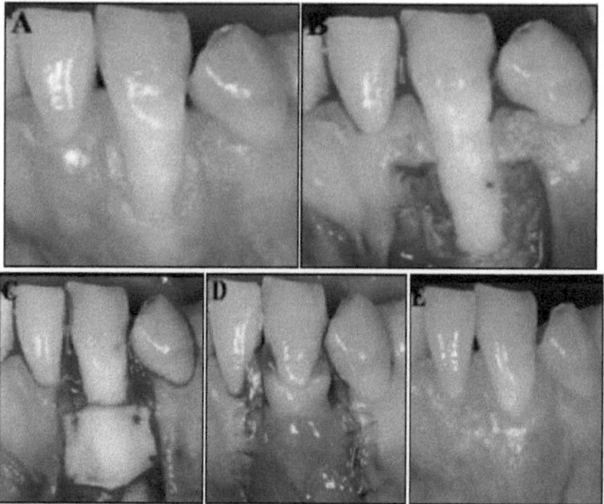

Figure 28: Treatment of gingival recession of a lower canine with a coronally advanced flap and connective tissue graft

(A) : Preoperative status(B): Full-thickness detachment

(C): Connective tissue graft taken from the palate sutured to the root face

(D) : Coronally advanced and sutured flap(E): 6-month healing with complete root coverage (44)

1.2.1. Benefits

G.T.C. offers a greater chance of success and predictability than free gingival grafting, as well as better aesthetic results.It acts as a biological filler, improving the adaptation and stability of the flap to the root during early wound repair, making the wound more resistant to damage.thicker gingival phenotype with greater potential to achieve complete root coverage with less pain in the donor area(44).

1.2.2. Disadvantages

This is a delicate technique that requires in-depth knowledge and assessment of the palatal donor site, as the risk of violating the neurovascular bundle when harvesting donor tissue, particularly when the palate is shallow, remains present throughout the harvest. It is difficult to perform in the presence of mucosal retraction, and the carries a higher risk of tissue perforation.It may sometimes require a 2-stage operation, and healing is by secondary intention, which leads to greater postoperative discomfort for the patient. (52)

1.2.3. Indications

G.T.G. is mainly indicated for root coverage, increasing peri-implant soft tissue thickness, masking discoloured roots, reconstructing the interdental papilla, peri-implant soft tissue dehiscence and increasing ridge height and width(44,53).

1.2.4. Protocol

1.2.4.1. sampling sites

Most studies describe two main sites:*The hard palate: A large C.T.G. (> 3 mm on average) can be harvested from the palate from the PM1 to the maxillary M2; the palate heals rapidly, thanks to its rich vascularisation, allowing a new harvest to be taken from the same site in a short space of time. However, there is a risk of severe post-operative pain, or even complications such as necrosis or infection, causing considerable discomfort (54).
The thickness of the palatal masticatory mucosa increases on average from the canine region (3.46 mm) to the premolar region (3.81 mm at PM2), then decreases in the M1 region (3.13 mm) before increasing again in the M2 region (3.39 mm). It also increases gradually from the marginal gingiva of the maxillary teeth towards the medial raphe of the palate. (54)

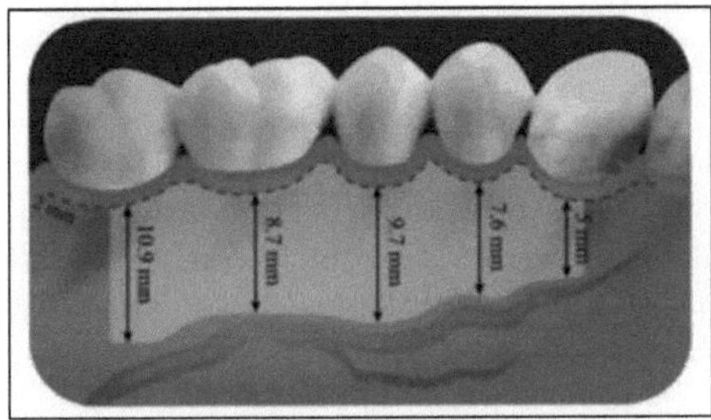

Figure 29: Schematic representation of the safety zone in patients with healthy periodontium(54)

*The maxillary tuberosity: This presents a promising alternative donor site to the palate for soft tissue harvesting, reducing patient morbidity, while containing more lamina propria, better collagen density and less submucosa than a C.T.G. harvested from the deep lateral palate, giving it better long-term dimensional stability. In terms of aesthetics, the results seem to be better with a graft taken from the palate rather than the tuberosity(44,54).
Other sites can be exploited, such as the edentulous ridge; this involves providing soft tissue of the same histological composition as the attached gingiva of the recipient site. The vestibule represents a new site for harvesting connective tissue, offering excellent aesthetic results, and causing less retraction of the graft because it is less fibrous than that of the palate or tuberosity(44,54).

1.2.4.2. Sampling techniques

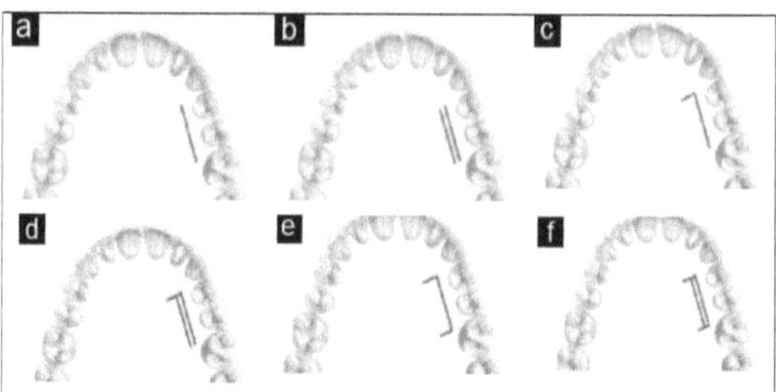

Figure 30: Liu and Weisgold classification of incisions

(a), (b): Class I type A and B (c), (d): Class II type A and B (d), (e) : Class III type A and B(55)

Various techniques for harvesting connective tissue grafts (CTG) have been described in the literature and their indications depend in particular on the quality of the palatal mucosa(55).
-In cases where the palatal thickness is sufficient : Traditional harvesting techniques such as the trap door, the single incision technique and parallel incisions have been proposed to obtain a palatal CTG.The main aim of these methods was to achieve first-line healing by preserving a primary palatal flap which was then sutured to the donor site after harvesting(44).
-If the palatal thickness is insufficient: There is a risk of incorporating fatty and glandular tissue into the graft, originating from the deep part of the connective tissue. This tissue must therefore be removed, as it may interfere with the revascularisation of the graft, leading to its necrosis. ☐ In such cases, a de-epithelialised free gingival graft technique was recommended. (55) Zucchelli et al(56) hypothesised that differences in the quality of the connective tissues used in the two techniques were responsible for this increase in gingival thickness because the de-epithelialised free gingival graft allows the portion of connective tissue closest to the epithelium to be incorporated into the graft. This tissue is dense, firmer, more stable and probably more suitable for root coverage.The de-epithelialised free gingival graft technique has been shown to be simple and applicable to a variety of clinical situations, with minimal morbidity and no post-operative complications(55).

1.2.4.3. Techniques associated with placement of the graft

Various techniques associated with GCE have been proposed. The graft can be buried under a partial thickness flap displaced more or less coronally, it can also be buried, either under a laterally displaced flap, or in an envelope prepared around the tissue deficit. (57)
Since a 2014 European consensus, the coronal tract flap (CTL) with connective tissue graft has been considered the gold standard for root overlays and for keratinised tissue gain in height and thickness. Due to unfavourable local anatomical conditions, LCT has been contraindicated in certain clinical situations.(58) Lateral flap: Zucchelli et al(59) evaluated the efficacy, in terms of root coverage, of a modified surgical approach to the laterally displaced flap procedure with a submarginal incision and a mixed thickness flap in the donor site, for

the treatment of gingival defects. They also suggested the coronal advancement of the laterally displaced flap. Specific characteristics of the keratinised tissue lateral to the defects were taken into account for the indication: lateral width of the keratinised tissue at least 6 mm greater than the width of the recession and lateral height of the donor keratinised tissue at least 2 mm greater than the buccal probing depth of the adjacent tooth or teeth(58).

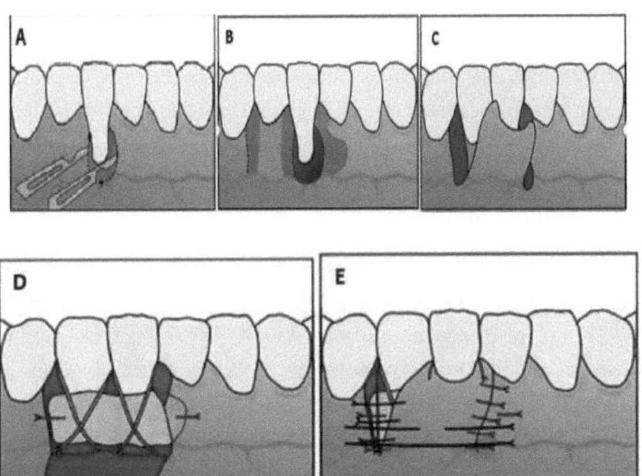

Figure 31: Schematic representation of the Zucchelli et al. technique(59)
(A) Internal and external bevel incision + intrasulcular

(B) Delineation of gingival thickness (purple: partial thickness, yellow:total thickness)(C):
Lateral flap placement
(D) : Placement of the graft
(E) Flap sutures(58)

Tunnelling: This is a minimally invasive periodontal plastic surgery technique. This technique offers a number of advantages, such as the absence of a vertical discharge incision; coronal displacement of the flap to cover as much of the connective tissue graft as possible, which increases the graft's survival rate; and improved blood supply, which means faster healing in the first instance, with less scarring and minimal trauma. (60)(61)

1.3. New perspectives

> **Laser :**

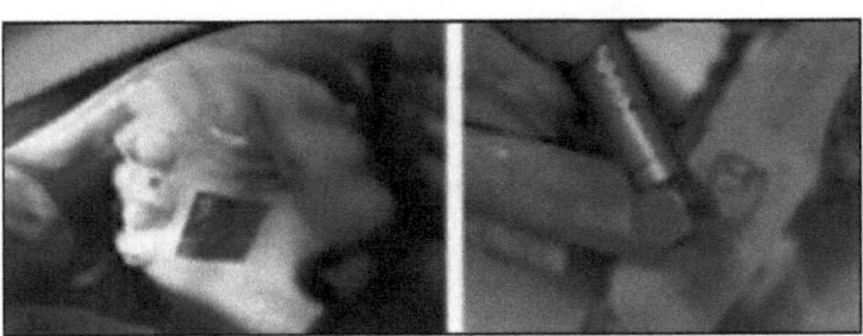

Figure 32: Preparation of a palatal donor site and laser trimming Er;Cr:YSGG (46)

➤ Laser as a sampling method :

Recently, the application of laser for oral surgery has attracted particular attention due to its advantages over conventional methods such as less pain, faster healing, coagulation conducted on a dry field for better visualisation. Laser technology with appropriate parameters has enabled tissue fusion and incision with better visual and mechanical access and less discomfort(46). Different wavelengths can be used for this purpose, including CO2, Er:YAG, Er;Cr:YSGG, diode and Nd:YAG lasers.The erbium family has shown advantages such as less thermal damage, the depth of penetration results in less trauma and makes the surgical process a comfortable experience for patients. The use of the laser instead of the scalpel showed a similar or even shorter healing time compared with the conventional method, with favourable wound healing and incorporation of the graft with no delay(46).

➤ Photobiomodulation and wound healing :

The development of a new blood supply between the graft and the recipient site plays an essential role in graft shrinkage. Thus, by accelerating collateral circulation of the periosteal bed and connective tissue, graft shrinkage is reduced. Low-level laser therapy (LLLT) has been successfully used for photobiomodulation and accelerated wound healing. These biostimulation and biomodulation effects are obtained by acting on the cellular mitochondrial respiratory chain or membrane potential. TLBN improves tissue neovascularisation and increases the proliferation, maturation and attachment of fibroblasts. It also has anti-inflammatory effects, so TLBN promotes analgesia, restores microcapillary circulation, normalises vascular wall permeability and reduces oedema.In the literature, although daily activation of TLBN has been recommended for the first week after surgery, there are also applications that are performed every 48 h for 1 week or every other day for 2 weeks (62).

➤ Hyaluronic acid :

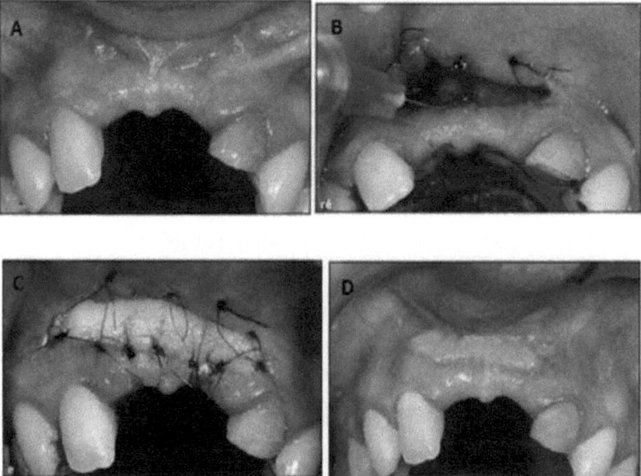

Figure 33: Use of HA in combination with a gingival graft

(A): Pre-operative status (B): Preparation of recipient site and application

of the HA (C): suture placement (D): post-operative status (after one month) (63)

Hyaluronic acid (HA) is a biomaterial that induces capillary proliferation and angiogenesis with its components increasing vascularisation after formation via biodegradation. It has previously been reported that the application of Hyaluronic acid prevents shrinkage of the skin graft and increases vascularisation. Studies carried out in 2020 by Turgut et al(63) showed that the use of hyaluronic acid enables the formation of a well-vascularised layer, and when applied locally to the recipient bed, it acts as a barrier against graft shrinkage between the recipient bed and the graft. Application of HA to the recipient bed as a thin layer accelerates vascularisation by providing additional revascularisation over its entire surface with the centre of the graft (63).

> **Cynoacrylate**

Cyanoacrylate adhesives have been widely used to close skin wounds and in a number of surgical procedures involving the skin, mucous membranes and various tissues, including those in the oral cavity.With the emergence of such chemical adhesives, and because of the interference of conventional sutures in the tissue healing process, some professionals have begun to replace sutures with these tissue adhesives.The main advantages of bioadhesive materials are their high tissue compatibility and long half-life; the presence of haemostatic, analgesic and antibacterial properties; a high potential for adhesion and biodegradation; and the ability to maintain the position/stabilisation of injured tissue. Cyanoacrylate appears to have analgesic effects and less pain when applied to the wound closure and covering the donor and recipient areas, thus reducing the need for post-operative analgesic medication; and has a healing effect in the closure of the donor area to the palate. In addition, it can reduce bleeding time after surgery and prevents late bleeding during the first post-operative week (64).

> **Ultrasound guidance :**

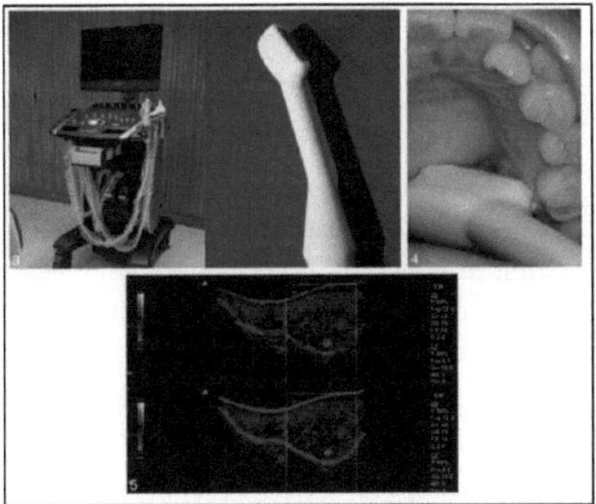

Figure 34: Doppler ultrasound image of the mucosa of the palate showing its thickness and the course of the greater palatine artery (65)

Ultrasound is widely used in the medical field for diagnoses involving the tissues of the human body. The probe must be in contact with the tissue in the target area as closely as possible.As a non-invasive method, ultrasound allows the thickness of the gum to be measured at several points and at different angles, which is useful for selecting the most appropriate donor site in relation to the gum at the recipient site.

However, no intra-oral probe for oral surgery has been specifically designed to adapt to the curves and soft mucosal area of the mouth, in particular the palatal vault(65).

2. Results and recovery clinical

Healing after soft tissue graft surgery goes through various stages and takes around two months.

After 10 days: Newly regenerated reddish tissue was observed at the recipient sites. Most sites grafted with FGG were slightly reddish, with a slightly pronounced contour. There were no apparent differences between the dental and implant sites.

After 30 days: Varying degrees of tissue maturation were observed. Recipient beds showed some shrinkage and apical scar-like linear tissue formation.

After 60 days: Tissue maturation and keratinisation appeared almost complete. Shrinkage of the recipient bed was more pronounced, whatever the treatment modality. A band of scar tissue was still discernible apically(66).

3. Complications

Mucogingival surgery techniques are not without complications. A distinction is made between early post-operative complications, which are the most frequently described, such as bleeding, pain or inflammation. Late complications, which appear a few weeks or even months or years after the treatment has been carried out, are rare.

3.1. Major complications

They are essentially represented by the epithelial cyst, which is a chronic inflammatory lesion partially or totally delimited by tissue, the cul-de-sac : invagination formation, with a probing depth greater than 0.5 mm, bone exostoses, superficial re-epithelialisation, which consists of partial or complete proliferation of the graft's original superficial epithelial layer, resulting in a mucosal surface similar to that of the donor area or superficial epithelial bands: epithelial tissue located on the graft without being adhered to it.

3.2. Complications minor

These include colour change, which is an aesthetic alteration in relation to the appearance of the surrounding tissues, or superficial revascularisation by the proliferation of multiple blood vessels modifying the superficial aesthetics of the graft(67) (68).

III. DENTIN GRAFT AUTOGENOUS

Extracted human teeth have long been regarded as infectious waste, and their alveoli are generally not treated for physiological healing.Advances in tissue engineering and stem cell science have led to the development of new bone regeneration techniques in the maxillofacial region. Dentin has been an important subject of study due to its potential use as a bone substitute(69) and the idea of its use for hard tissue augmentation is considered a logical recent alternative to autogenous bone(70).

In 2010, Kim et al (71) described the first ever use of dentine in implant dentistry, obtaining dentine from the patient's extracted teeth(72).

1. Properties of dentine

Autogenous dentine has ideal physical properties (density, roughness and homogeneity) and chemical properties (composed of calcium/phosphate similar to human bone in the cortex)(72). Root dentin is considered to be an ideal bioactive material for hard tissue regeneration, it has low crystallinity and a higher percentage of other organic materials, and can therefore be suitable as a bone graft compared to the crown part, its inorganic and organic composition is relatively similar to natural bone which minimises the reaction to foreign bodies due to the genetic homogeneity proving its biocompatibility.(70) (73) (69)Human dentin is made up of 70% organic matter with four types of calcium phosphate (hydroxyapatite, tricalcium phosphate, octacalcium phosphate and amorphous calcium phosphate), which give dentin its **osteo-conductive** properties. The hydroxyapatite in dentin is in the form of low-crystalline calcium phosphate, which makes it easily degradable by the activity of osteoclasts. It is composed of 20% organic matter, of which 90 % type I collagen network and 10% non-collagen proteins (osteo-calcine),osteo-nectin, sialoprotein and phosphoprotein, which are involved in bone calcification) and growth factors (bone morphogenetic proteins: BMP, and insulin-like growth factor, which give the tooth **osteo-inductive** properties); the remaining 10% is water (72).

2. Techniques

Two possible applications for the use of dentin graft as a bone substitute have been proposed. One is its use as a graft requiring processing via demineralisation procedures similar to those used in allogeneic bone manipulation. The other is in the form of fresh autologous material, in which dentine is used without prior demineralisation. This second alternative can be used in particle or block form(69).

2.1. Fresh dentine: Block dentine technique

Dental roots have been shown in various clinical and radiographic studies to be an alternative to autogenous bone.

2.1.1. Operating protocol

The extracted tooth is first treated to remove all debris, calculus and the cementum layer exposing the underlying dentin (a straight burr is used to remove the cementum under copious irrigation): removing the cementum layer will improve the ankylosis between the graft and the defect site. The graft is then cut and shaped according to the defect site on the chair for a few minutes immediately after extraction of the tooth, to fit very close to the recipient bone.

The tooth root block was immersed in dentin cleaning solution followed by saline buffer solution to obtain a graft free of all organic debris, resulting in a sterile bacteria-free graft.

This was followed by stabilisation of the prepared tooth root graft with titanium screws (mini-screws with a minimum diameter of preferably 1.2 mm to fix the tooth root to the underlying bone) to stabilise the graft to avoid any micromovement that could impede graft healing.(73,74)

2.1.2. Results

Postoperative **clinical and radiographic** ridge width at 6 months was significantly greater than baseline suggesting a definite gain in ridge width.
Histological analysis of the bone crest obtained :

▪ 24 weeks after augmentation, the root of the tooth was firmly adherent to the native bone, which has already been proven by experimental studies that basal ankylosis exists (70).
▪ Six months later, there was operational formation of new, organised native bone. No remnants of the dental block graft were observed: the graft block was completely resorbed and replaced by non-mineralised tissue which was replaced by woven bone(73,75).

2.1.3. Comparison with autogenous bone

Schwarz and colleagues(76) conducted a study comparing autogenous tooth roots with autogenous bone blocks for lateral alveolar ridge augmentation followed by implant placement in two stages. They observed no statistical difference in crest width after 6 months between 2 groups as both allowed successful implant placement(73).
Although it does not have the osteogenic capacity of autogenous bone and its quantity is also limited, the use of autogenous dentine as a grafting material has a positive effect and avoids the morbidity and complications associated with autogenous bone harvesting(72).

2.1.4. Benefits

Dentine grafting offers a number of advantages: as it is an autograft, there is no possibility of graft rejection or cross-infection; the graft is the extracted tooth itself, so there is no second surgical site; and healing is associated with the integration of the graft with the basal bone and the gradual resorption of the graft and replacement by a new, viable graft. This type of planning saves the patient a great deal of time and money and considerably improves the dimensions of the residual ridge without any additional material(73,74).
High mechanical strength is another advantage of mechanically unchanged dentine, which allows primary stability of the implant (70).

2.1.5. Disadvantages

Complete integration takes about 6 months. This time could have been reduced if the block had been demineralised or perforated(73).

2.1.6. Complications

The en bloc technique risks exposure of the graft, which can be avoided by rigorous selection of cases with a good tissue biotype, or infection, which can be avoided by good instrumentation of the extracted root surface. Care must be taken to avoid pseudarthrosis of the graft(73,75).

2.1.7. Limits

The indication for this technique is limited by the infrequent presence of a healthy tooth root without caries and restorations. In fact, the selection of cases is very specific and must be such that only one bone cortex is missing and that the buccal or palatal cortex is present to support the graft and ensure good vascularisation(73,74).

2.2. Fresh dentine: Particulate dentine technique :

The **SDG (Smart Dentin Grinder®)** procedure prepares dentin into bacteria-free particles using freshly extracted autologous teeth, ready for immediate use as biomaterials(69). This machine is designed to crush and sort extracted teeth into dental particles of specific sizes(70).

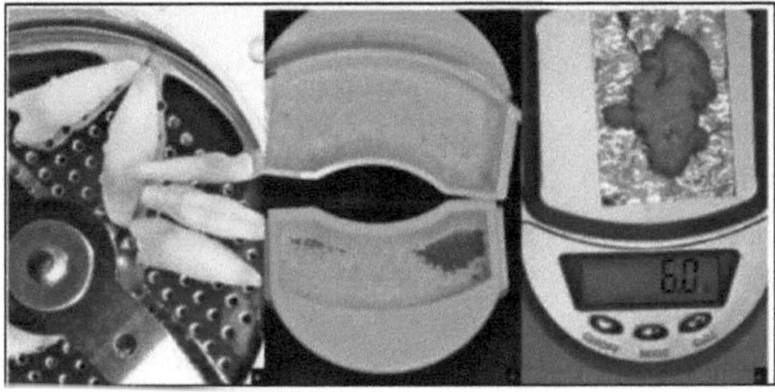

Figure 35: Preparation of dentine by SDGTeeth in the SDG chamber (b) Particles of different sizes from 300 to 1200

μm (c) particle weight (77)

2.2.1. Operating protocol

The particulate dental graft is prepared immediately after tooth extraction (70):
- Tooth extraction: Extractions were carried out in a non-traumatic manner using manual syndesmotomes or piezosurgery to avoid damage to the alveolar ridge at the time of extraction. A complete alveolar curettage was then performed.
- Preparation and processing of the dental material: Once the dental material had been obtained and used as an alveolar filling material in selected cases, the preparation and processing of the material was carried out as described below:
1. Use of tungsten carbide flame or fissure burs: removal of crowns or fillings of any kind (composite resins or amalgams), caries or discolouration of dentine, the periodontal ligament and/or dental plaque.
2. Rinse with sterile physiological saline and then dry with an air syringe.

3. The dentin fragments are ground in a grinding chamber capable of crushing the roots into particles of 300 and 1200 microns. The particles were ground using vibrations for 20 seconds. All particles smaller than 300 microns were rejected.
4. The particulate material obtained was soaked for 10 minutes in a glass container sterilised with 0.5 molar NaOH with 20% ethanol. This process dissolves the organic residues, bacteria and toxins present in the dentine.

5. Washing in sterile saline solution blocked with phosphate(69).

2.2.2. Results

Clinical results after application of dental roots or demineralised dentin matrix have shown acceptable clinical and radiographic results(70)

2.2.3. Indications

This method is indicated for horizontal or vertical ridge augmentation, preservation of the extraction socket, aesthetic restoration of the alveolar bone or perforated sinus membrane and improvement of initial implant stabilisation(70).

2.2.4. Benefits

Fresh particulate grafting preserves the tooth in particulate form without diminishing the bioactive properties of the dentin: like a **biocompatible, bioactive** and **bio-inerte** graft. It allows us to prepare a natural biomaterial from freshly extracted autologous teeth in the form of a bacteria-free particle for immediate use as an autogenous graft biomaterial in a single surgical session.(77)
These particles contain proteins similar in weight to the bone morphogenetic proteins (BMPs) abundant in tooth substance(69).

2.2.5. Limits

In cases where the extracted tooth has undergone root canal treatment, this has not been used as a donor material(69).

2.3. Demineralised dentine

In recent years, chemical modification, in particular demineralisation, has been considered an essential element: an initial step in the application of dentine prior to grafting(78).
The demineralisation of dentine results in the elimination of most of the mineral phase and immunogenic components, while retaining a very small fraction of minerals and most of the type I collagen, thus providing an osteoconductive and osteoinductive scaffold containing several growth factors(79).Demineralised dentine is currently available in two forms: powder and block. The importance of its geometry has already been highlighted by many researchers.
Demineralised dentine powder is usually mixed with other suitable materials (such as hydroxypropylcellulose) to form a paste that can be easily moulded at the site of the bone defect.A block of demineralised dentin is made from the root cut at the cemento-enamel junction. The artificial macropores that run through it have a diameter of around 300 to 400 µm. Such porosity can influence the osteoconductive characteristics of the scaffold by creating spaces for the attachment, differentiation and growth of osteoblasts and vascular invasion from surrounding tissues. This will contribute to active bone growth in critically sized bone defects(79).

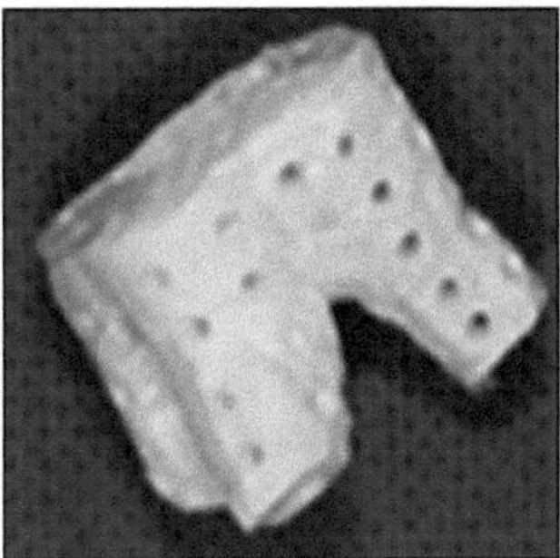

Figure 36: Demineralised dentine block with micropores (300-400μm) (79).

2.3.1. Operating protocol

1- The extracted teeth are cleaned of soft tissue and any restorative material.
2- They were then ground to obtain refined dentin particles with a diameter of approximately
1 mm. The dentin particles were partially demineralised in 2% HNO3 and rinsed in 0.1 M
Tris-HCl (pH 7.4).
This operation is performed during the bone augmentation operation(80).

2.3.2. Results

The quantity and quality of the new bone formation according to the histomorphometric study
showed favourable results. Based on the current results, autogenous dental graft material has a
clinical efficacy comparable to that of inorganic bovine bone material and appears to be a
viable option.particularly in cases where dental extraction and immediate augmentation of the
alveolar bone are required(81).

2.3.3. Benefits

The autogenous origin and favourable clinical results showed that these materials offer good
osteoinductive capabilities. Demineralised dentin granules independently induce bone and
cartilage formation, and the bone induction sequence was similar to that of demineralised
bone matrix. Excellent osteo-conductive healing capacity in critically sized defects and bone
remodelling capabilities that could be attributed to its minerals, such as Hydoxyl-apatite and
TCP. (77)(79)No infections were observed in studies carried out on demineralised dentine.
This could be explained by the fact that demineralisation is effective for antimicrobial
activity(82).

2.3.4. Indications

The use of demineralised dentine is indicated for guided bone regeneration, sinus bone
grafting (ROG) using demineralised dentine powder, alveolar preservation: limiting post-
extraction resorption or ridge augmentation(79).

2.3.5. Limits

As demineralisation is a complicated and time-consuming process, extracted teeth have to be sent to other institutes for preparation, resulting in a prolonged treatment time . In most clinical studies using dentine matrix, approximately 12 hours (overnight) were required for dentine demineralisation (78) .
Although demineralised dentine has matrix-derived growth and differentiation factors for efficient osteogenesis, the newly formed bone that is generated and the residual demineralised dentine are too weak to allow adequate implant anchorage(77).

2.4. Dental shell technique

This technique is a modification of the bone shell technique. (83) Autogenous dentin, harvested from impacted molars, was cut into thin shells (≤ 2 mm) and fixed to the recipient site. The space between the dentin shells and the residual bone was filled with either bone, dentin or alloplastic mineral particles(78).

2.4.1. Operating protocol

1- The technique used to prepare the dentine graft is a commercially available technology consisting of a grinder for dentine particulation and substances for disinfection and demineralisation(83).
The partial demineralisation of dentine, which was achieved using a 10% EDTA solution, is able to promote replacement resorption and new bone formation due to the exposure of the collagen network and the release of osteogenic growth factors, such as bone morphogenetics. proteins.(83)
2- The non-demineralised dentine shells used can be prepared in the chair in just 30 minutes.
3- The grafting procedure was carried out in a surgery immediately after the extraction of a tooth.

2.4.2. Results

The histological results showed new bone formation on the outer and inner surfaces of the dentine envelope, suggesting the osteoconductive and even osteoinductive capacities of dentine(78).

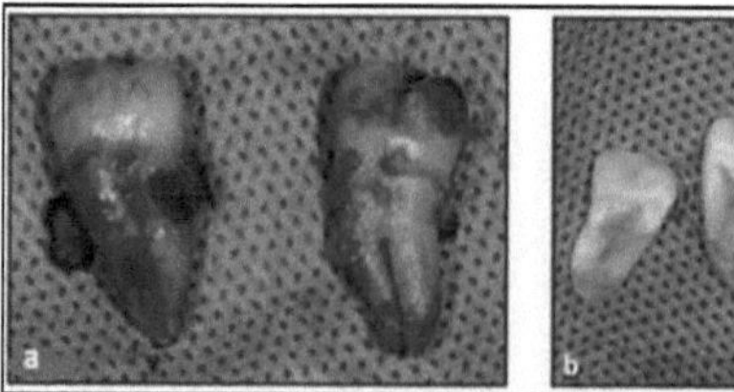

Figure 37: Preparation of dentine shells Extracted wisdom teeth Blocks of dentine shaped into thin shells < 2mm (78)

2.4.3. Benefits

Particulate dentine in the space between the bone and the dentine shell leads to better revascularisation and regeneration than a procedure using solid blocks of dentine and has significantly less graft resorption than autogenous bone grafts(84). Although teeth in contact with the oral cavity were used for grafting, no increase in inflammation was observed histologically, and there was no increase in the rate of wound infection or graft loss.Bone harvesting and the resulting possible donor site morbidity can be avoided, resulting in a low complication rate with a high success prognosis, and thanks to the chemical treatment and disinfection that can be carried out, the dental material can be prepared for storage and preserved for future use(84)(83). This technique combines the stability of cortical bone grafts with improved osteo-conductive properties. It guarantees a stable scaffold will be created by the thin shell, which is rigidly fixed at a distance.(83)

2.4.4. Indications

For lateral ridge augmentation: a greater horizontal deficit can be increased(83)

2.4.5. Limits

It cannot be indicated if the tooth to be replaced is no longer present and there are no other non-conservable teeth, or in the case of major defects of the alveolar ridge(84). Large-scale bone defects that extend beyond the space occupied by the dentine shells can be maintained and can also be excluded from this treatment(78).

CONCLUSION

Treatments aimed at increasing bone and gum volume are becoming increasingly common in oral surgery, and should be guided by the prosthetic plan initially drawn up, taking into account the patient's age and the age of the prosthesis.bone and gingival morphology and general patient factors.This book has detailed the different techniques for autogenous bone grafts, either block or particulate, harvested from extra-oral or intra-oral sites and placed using several procedures.It also highlighted the types of connective and epithelial gingival grafts and the use of dentine in its various forms as a bone substitute. We also shed light on certain new technologies that are emerging and could improve the success rate or broaden the fields of application of these techniques.Compared with all xeno- and allograft procedures, autogenous materials have proven to be superior from a biological, immunological and even medico-legal point of view. This is why most surgeons and researchers are increasingly interested in this type of rehabilitation.

REFERENCES

1. Aloy-Prosper A, Penarrocha-Oltra D, Penarrocha-Diago Ma, Penarrocha-Diago M. The outcome of intraoral onlay block bone grafts on alveolar ridge augmentations: A systematic review. Med Oral Patol Oral Cirugia Bucal. 2015;e251-8.
2. Zhao X, Zou L, Chen Y, Tang Z. Staged horizontal bone augmentation for dental implants in aesthetic zones: A prospective randomized controlled clinical trial comparing a half-columnar bone block harvested from the ramus versus a rectangular bone block from the symphysis. Int J Oral Maxillofac Surg. Oct 2020;49(10):1326-34.
3. Novy LFS, Aguiar EG, de Arruda JAA, de Castro MAA, Moreira AN, dos Santos EG, et al. Linear and volumetric gain after vertical bone augmentation in the posterior mandible using an autologous cortical tenting method. Int J Oral Maxillofac Surg. nov 2019;48(11):1485-91.
4. Schmidt AH. Autologous bone graft: Is it still the gold standard? Injury, Elsevier, June 2021
5. Suda, A.J., Schamberger, C.T. & Viergutz, T. Donor site complications following anterior iliac crest bone graft for treatment of distal radius fractures. Arch Orthop Trauma Surg 139, 423-428 (2019). https://doi.org/10.1007/s00402-018-3098-3
6. Yuce M, Adali E, Turk G, Isik G, Gunbay T. Three-dimensional bone grafting in dental implantology using autogenous bone ring transplant: Clinical outcomes of a one-stage technique. Niger J Clin Pract. 2019;22(7):977.
7. Aswin Beck, Dirk Nehrbass, Martin J. Stoddart, Damiano Schiuma, Jim Green, Jennifer L. Lansdowne, R. Geoff Richards, Ludovic P. Bouré,_The use of Reamer Irrigator Aspirator (RIA) autograft harvest in the treatment of critical-sized iliac wing defects in sheep: Investigation of dexamethasone and beta-tricalcium phosphate augmentation, Bone, Volume 53, Issue 2, 2013
8. Starch-Jensen T, Deluiz D, Deb S, Bruun NH, Tinoco EMB. Harvesting of Autogenous Bone Graft from the Ascending Mandibular Ramus Compared with the Chin Region: a Systematic Review and Meta-Analysis Focusing on Complications and Donor Site Morbidity. J Oral Maxillofac

9. Kim R, Sokoya M, Ducic Y, Williams F. Free-Flap Reconstruction of the Mandible. Semin Plast Surg. Feb 2019;33(01):046-53.

10. Ducic Y, Defatta R, Wolfswinkel EM, Weathers WM, Hollier LH Jr. Tunneling technique for expedited fibula free tissue harvest. Craniomaxillofac Trauma Reconstr. 2013;6(4):233-236. doi:10.1055/s-0033-1349208
11. Fernandes RP, Yetzer JG. Reconstruction of acquired oromandibular defects. Oral Maxillofac Surg Clin North Am. 2013 May;25(2):241-9. doi: 10.1016/j.coms.2013.02.003.
12. Imamura E, Mayahara M, Inoue S, Miyamoto M, Funae T, Watanabe Y, et al. Trabecular structure and composition analysis of human autogenous bone donor sites using micro-computed tomography. J Oral Biosci. March 2021;63(1):74-9.
13. Nicot R, Schlund M, Touzet-Roumazeille S, Ferri J, Raoul G. Unicortical Calvarial Autologous Bone Graft Harvest. Plast Reconstr Surg - Glob Open. Nov 2020;8(11):e3241.
14. Ritschl LM, Fichter AM, Grill FD, Hart D, Hapfelmeier A, Deppe H, et al. Bone volume

change following vascularized free bone flap reconstruction of the mandible. J Cranio-Maxillofac Surg. Sept 2020;48(9):859-67.

15. Wilkman T, Apajalahti S, Wilkman E, Törnwall J, Lassus P. A Comparison of Bone Resorption Over Time: An Analysis of the Free Scapular, Iliac Crest, and Fibular Microvascular Flaps in Mandibular Reconstruction. J Oral Maxillofac Surg. March 1, 2017;75(3):616-21.

16. Chen S-H, Chen H-C, Horng S-Y, Tai H-C, Hsieh J-H, Yeong E-K, et al. Reconstruction for Osteoradionecrosis of the Mandible: Superiority of Free Iliac Bone Flap to Fibula Flap in Postoperative Infection and Healing. Ann Plast Surg. Sep 2014;73:S18.

17. Kilinc A, Saruhan N, Ertas U, Korkmaz IH, Kaymaz I. An Analysis of Mandibular Symphyseal Graft Sufficiency for Alveolar Cleft Bone Grafting. J Craniofac Surg. jan 2017;28(1):147-50.

18. Shirzadeh A, Rahpeyma A, Khajehahmadi S. A Prospective Study of Chin Bone Graft Harvesting for Unilateral Maxillary Alveolar Cleft During Mixed Dentition. J Oral Maxillofac Surg. Jan 2018;76(1):180-8.

19. Clavero J, Lundgren S. Ramus or Chin Grafts for Maxillary Sinus Inlay and Local Onlay Augmentation: Comparison of Donor Site Morbidity and Complications. Clin Implant Dent Relat Res. Oct 2003;5(3):154-60.

20. Khoury F, Hanser T. Mandibular Bone Block Harvesting from the Retromolar Region: A 10-Year Prospective Clinical Study. Int J Oral Maxillofac Implants. May 2015;30(3):688-97.

21. Verdugo F, Simonian K, McDonald RS, Nowzari H. Quantitation of Mandibular Ramus Volume as a Source of Bone Grafting. Clin Implant Dent Relat Res. Oct 2009;11:e32-7.

22. Ataman-Duruel E, Duruel O, Nares S, Stanford C, Tözüm T. Quantity and Quality of Intraoral Autogenous Block Graft Donor Sites with Cone Beam Computed Tomography. Int J Oral Maxillofac Implants. July 2020;35(4):782-8.

23. Thomas Belloir. Retro-incisal palatal bone harvesting: a feasibility study. Human Medicine and Pathology. 2017. ffdumas-01503933e

24. El Zahwy M, Taha SA allah K, Mounir R, Mounir M. Assessment of vertical ridge augmentation and marginal bone loss using autogenous onlay vs inlay grafting techniques with simultaneous implant placement in the anterior maxillary esthetic zone: A randomized clinical trial. Clin Implant Dent Relat Res. Dec 2019;21(6):1140-7.

25. Modabber A, Legros C, Rana M, Gerressen M, Riediger D, Ghassemi A. Evaluation of computer-assisted jaw reconstruction with free vascularized fibular flap compared to conventional surgery: a clinical pilot study. Int J Med Robot. 2012 Jun;8(2):215-20. doi: 10.1002/rcs.456. Epub 2011 Dec 30.

26. Prevost A, Delanoe F, Cavallier Z, Muller S, Lopez R, Lauwers F. Surgical benefit of mandibular morphometric analysis: A new tool to standardize mandibular reconstruction. Giuliani A, editor. PLOS ONE. 6 Nov 2020;15(11):e0240558.

27. Chandra R, Shivateja K, Reddy A. Autogenous Bone Ring Transplant vs Autologous Growth Factor-Enriched Bone Graft Matrix in Extraction Sockets with Deficient Buccal Bone: A Comparative Clinical Study. Int J Oral Maxillofac Implants. Nov 2019;34(6):1424-33.

28. Perez PI, Sloneker DR, Bloom AG, Vincent AG, Hohman MH, Harsha WJ, et al. Non-vascularized Fibular Cortex Grafts with Osteocutaneous Free Fibula Transfer: A Novel

Technique in Midface Reconstruction. Ann Otol Rhinol Laryngol. 23 Nov 2020;000348942097273.

29. Adrien Paul. Bone grafts in oral surgery: new perspectives. Human medicine and pathology. 2014. ffdumas-01016817e

30. Deshpande S, Deshmukh J, Deshpande S, Khatri R, Deshpande S. Vertical and horizontal ridge augmentation in anterior maxilla using autograft, xenograft and titanium mesh with simultaneous placement of endosseous implants. J Indian Soc Periodontol. 9 Jan 2014;18(5):661.

31. Rachmiel A, Emodi O, Rachmiel D, Israel Y, Shilo D. Sandwich osteotomy for the reconstruction of deficient alveolar bone. Int J Oral Maxillofac Surg. Oct 2018;47(10):1350-7.

32. Cortellini P, Pini Prato G, Tonetti MS. Periodontal regeneration of human infrabony defects. II. Re-entry procedures and bone measures. J Periodontol. Apr 1993;64(4):261-8.

33. Atef M, Osman AH, Hakam M. Autogenous interpositional block graft vs onlay graft for horizontal ridge augmentation in the mandible. Clin Implant Dent Relat Res. August 2019;21(4):678-85.

34. Pourdanesh F, Esmaeelinejad M, Aghdashi F. Clinical outcomes of dental implants after use of tenting for bony augmentation: a systematic review. Br J Oral Maxillofac Surg. dec 2017;55(10):999-1007.

35. Khojasteh A, Esmaeelinejad M, Aghdashi F. Regenerative Techniques in Oral and Maxillofacial Bone Grafting. A Textbook of Advanced Oral and Maxillofacial Surgery Volume 2.

36. Gregory R. Caldwell, DDS, MS/Michael P. Mills, DMD, MS/Richard Finlayson, DDS/Brian L. Mealey, DDS, MS Lateral Alveolar Ridge Augmentation Using Tenting Screws, Acellular Dermal Matrix, and Freeze-Dried Bone Allograft Alone or with Particulate Autogenous Bone PMID: 25734709; DOI: 10.11607/prd.2260

37. Le B, Burstein J, Sedghizadeh PP. Cortical tenting grafting technique in the severely atrophic alveolar ridge for implant site preparation. Implant Dent. March 2008;17(1):40-50.

38. Khoury, Fouad and Khoury, Charles. Mandibular bone block grafts: diagnosis, instrumentation, harvesting techniques and surgical procedures. Bone augmentation in oral implantology. Berlin: Quintessence, 2007.

39. Liang C, Lin X, Wang S-L, Guo L-H, Wang X-Y, Li J. Osteogenic potential of three different autogenous bone particles harvested during implant surgery. Oral Dis. Nov 2017;23(8):1099-108.

40. Coyac BR, Salvi G, Leahy B, Li Z, Salmon B, Hoffmann W, et al. A novel system exploits bone debris for implant osseointegration. J Periodontol. 10 Sep 2020;JPER.20-0099.

41. Younger, Edward M.; Chapman, Michael W. Morbidity at Bone Graft Donor Sites, Journal of Orthopaedic Trauma: September 1989 - Volume 3 - Issue 3 - p 192- 195

42. Flierl, M.A., Smith, W.R., Mauffrey, C. et al. Outcomes and complication rates of different bone grafting modalities in long bone fracture nonunions: a retrospective cohort study in 182 patients. J Orthop Surg Res 8, 33 (2013). https://doi.org/10.1186/1749-799X-8-33

43. Deramo P, Rose J. Flaps, Muscle And Musculocutaneous [Updated 2021 Jul 18]. In: StatPearls. Treasure Island (FL): StatPearls Publishing; 2021 Jan-.

44. Zucchelli G, Tavelli L, McGuire MK, Rasperini G, Feinberg SE, Wang H, et al. Autogenous soft tissue grafting for periodontal and peri-implant plastic surgical

reconstruction. J Periodontol. Jan 2020;91(1):9-16.

45. Scheyer ET, Sanz M, Dibart S, Greenwell H, John V, Kim DM, et al. Periodontal soft tissue non-root coverage procedures: a consensus report from the AAP Regeneration Workshop. J Periodontol. Feb 2015;86(2 Suppl):S73-76.

46. Fekrazad R, Chiniforush N, Kalhori K. All done procedure by laser in free gingival graft treatment: A case series study. J Cosmet Laser Ther. Jan 2, 2019;21(1):4-10.

47. Goyal L, AIIMS RISHIKESH, Gupta ND, DEPARTMENT OF PERIODONTICS AND COMMUNITY DENTISTRY, Gupta N, DEPARTMENT OF PERIODONTICS AND COMMUNITY DENTISTRY, Gupta N, DEPARTMENT OF PERIODONTICS AND COMMUNITY DENTISTRY
COMMUNITY DENTISTRY, et al. Free Gingival Graft as a Single Step Procedure for Treatment of Mandibular Miller Class I and II Recession Defects. WORLD J Plast Surg. Jan 1, 2019;8(1):12-7.

48. Cevallos CAR, de Resende DRB, Damante CA, Sant'Ana ACP, de Rezende MLR, Greghi SLA, et al. Free gingival graft and acellular dermal matrix for gingival augmentation: a 15-year clinical study. Clin Oral Investig. March 2020;24(3):1197-203.

49. Cortellini P, Pini Prato G. Coronally advanced flap and combination therapy for root coverage. Clinical strategies based on scientific evidence and clinical experience. Periodontol 2000. June 2012;59(1):158-84.

50. Miller PD. Root coverage using the free soft tissue autograft following citric acid application. III. A successful and predictable procedure in areas of deep-wide recession. Int J Periodontics Restorative Dent. 1985;5(2):14-37.

51. Bernimoulin JP, Lüscher B, Mühlemann HR. Coronally repositioned periodontal flap. Clinical evaluation after one year. J Clin Periodontol. Feb 1975;2(1):1-13.

52. Puri K, Kumar A, Khatri M, Bansal M, Rehan Mohd, Siddeshappa ST. 44-year journey of palatal connective tissue graft harvest: A narrative review. J Indian Soc Periodontol. 2019;23(5):395-408.

53. Giannobile, WV, Jung, RE, Schwarz, F; on behalf of the Groups of the 2nd Osteology Foundation Consensus Meeting. Evidence-based knowledge on the aesthetics and maintenance of peri-implant soft tissues: Osteology Foundation Consensus Report Part 1- Effects of Soft Tissue Augmentation Procedures on the Maintenance of Peri-implant Soft Tissue Health. Clin Oral Impl Res. 2018; 29(Suppl. 15): 7- 10. https://doi.org/10.1111/clr.13110

54. Morgane Valdenaire. Palatal connective tissue sampling: techniques and morbidity management. Life Sciences [q-bio]. 2020. ffhal-03298275e

55. Azar EL, Rojas MA, Patricia M, Carranza N. Histologic and Histomorphometric Analyses of De-epithelialized Free Gingival Graft in Humans. Restorative Dent. 2019;39(2):7.

56. Zucchelli G, Mele M, Stefanini M, Mazzotti C, Marzadori M, Montebugnoli L, et al. Patient morbidity and root coverage outcome after subepithelial connective tissue and de-epithelialized grafts: a comparative randomized-controlled clinical trial: Patient morbidity and root coverage outcome after grafts. J Clin Periodontol. 24 June 2010;no-no.

57. Erraji S, Ismaili Z, Ennibi OK. Buried connective tissue grafting: how to improve recovery predictability? Actual Odonto-Stomatol. March 2014;(267):35-9.

58. Bosco AF, de Almeida JM, Retamal-Valdes B, Tavares R, Latimer JM, Messina D, et al.

Laterally Positioned Flap with Subepithelial Connective Tissue Graft Modified One-Stage Procedure for the Treatment of Deep Isolated Gingival Recessions in Mandibular Incisors. Case Rep Dent. August 5, 2021;2021:2326152.

59. Zucchelli G, Cesari C, Amore C, Montebugnoli L, De Sanctis M. Laterally moved, coronally advanced flap: a modified surgical approach for isolated recession-type defects. J Periodontol. 2004 Dec;75(12):1734-41. doi: 10.1902/jop.2004.75.12.1734. Erratum in: J Periodontol. 2005 Aug;76(8):1425. PMID: 15732880.

60. Karmon B, Tavelli L, Rasperini G. Tunnel Technique with a Subperiosteal Bag for Horizontal Ridge Augmentation. Int J Periodontics Restorative Dent. March 2020;40(2):223-30.

61. Tözüm TF. A Promising Periodontal Procedure for the Treatment of Adjacent Gingival Recession Defects. J Can Dent Assoc. 2003;69(3):5.

62. Yildiz MS, Gunpinar S. Free gingival graft adjunct with low-level laser therapy: a randomized placebo-controlled parallel group study. Clin Oral Investig. Apr 2019;23(4):1845-54.

63. Çankaya ZT, Gürbüz S, Bakirarar B, Kurtis B. Evaluation of the Effect of Hyaluronic Acid Application on the Vascularization of Free Gingival Graft for Both Donor and Recipient Sites with Laser Doppler Flowmetry: A Randomized, Examiner-Blinded, Controlled Clinical Trial. Restorative Dent. 2020;40(2):12.

64. Veríssimo AH, Ribeiro AKC, Martins ARL de A, Gurgel BC de V, Lins RDAU. Comparative analysis of the hemostatic, analgesic and healing effects of cyanoacrylate on free gingival graft surgical wounds in donor and recipient areas: a systematic review. J Mater Sci Mater Med. Sept 2021;32(9):98.

65. Lee K-H, Jeong H-G, Kwak E-J, Park W, Kim K-D. Ultrasound Guided Free Gingival Graft: Case Report. J Oral Implantol. 2018 Oct 1;44(5):385-8.

66. Thoma DS, Lim H, Paeng K, Kim MJ, Jung RE, Hämmerle CHF, et al. Augmentation of keratinized tissue at tooth and implant sites by using autogenous grafts and collagen-based soft-tissue substitutes. J Clin Periodontol. Jan 2020;47(1):64-71.

67. Ripoll S, Fernández de Velasco-Tarilonte Á, Bullón B, Ríos-Carrasco B, Fernández-Palacín A. Complications in the Use of Deepithelialized Free Gingival Graft vs. Connective Tissue Graft: A One-Year Randomized Clinical Trial. Int J Environ Res Public Health. 23 Apr 2021;18(9):4504.

68. Curtis JW, McLain JB, Hutchinson RA. The incidence and severity of complications and pain following periodontal surgery. J Periodontol. Oct 1985;56(10):597-601.

69. del Canto-Diaz A, de Elio-Oliveros J, del Canto-Diaz M, Alobera-Gracia M, del Canto-Pingarron M, Martinez-Gonzalez J. Use of autologous tooth-derived graft material in the post-extraction dental socket. Pilot study. Med Oral Patol Oral Cirugia Bucal. 2018;0-0.

70. Elraee L, Moussa M, Adel-Khattab D. Autogenous Dentin Block of A Non Restorable Wisdom Tooth for Localized Horizontal Ridge Augmentation: Radiographic and Histological Analysis: A Preliminary Case Report. Clin Adv Periodontics. 5 Nov 2020;cap.10130.

71. Kim Y-K, Kim S-G, Byeon J-H, Lee H-J, Um I-U, Lim S-C, et al. Development of a novel bone grafting material using autogenous teeth. Oral Surg Oral Med Oral Pathol Oral Radiol Endod. 1 Apr 2010;109(4):496-503.

72. Sánchez-Labrador L, Martín-Ares M, Ortega-Aranegui R, López-Quiles J, Martínez-González JM. Autogenous Dentin Graft in Bone Defects after Lower Third Molar Extraction: A Split-Mouth Clinical Trial. Materials. 10 Jul 2020;13(14):3090.

73. Jana S, Thomas R, Kumar T, Shah R, Mehta DS, V GG. Immediate Ridge Augmentation Using Autogenous Tooth Root as a Block Graft in a Periodontally Hopeless Extraction Site: A Pilot Study. J Oral Implantol. Dec 9, 2019;0000-0000.

74. Yang K-I, Cho A-Y, Yang J-Y, Shin H-I, Lee W-P, Kim B-O, et al. Effect of autogenous tooth bone graft with membrane on Class II furcation defects in dogs: A histologic and histomorphometric study. Oral Biol Res. March 31, 2018;42(1):25-36.

75. Schwarz F, Golubovic V, Mihatovic I, Becker J. Periodontally diseased tooth roots used for lateral alveolar ridge augmentation. A proof-of-concept study. J Clin Periodontol. Sep 2016;43(9):797-803.

76. Schwarz F, Golubovic V, Becker K, Mihatovic I. Extracted tooth roots used for lateral alveolar ridge augmentation: a proof-of-concept study. J Clin Periodontol. Apr 2016;43(4):345-53.

77. Calvo-Guirado JL, Ballester-Montilla A, N De Aza P, Fernández-Domínguez M, Alexandre Gehrke S, Cegarra-Del Pino P, et al. Particulated, Extracted Human Teeth Characterization by SEM-EDX Evaluation as a Biomaterial for Socket Preservation: An in vitro Study. Materials. 25 Jan 2019;12(3):380.

78. Welan xiao, Chen Hu, Cenyu Chu, Yi Man. Autogenous dentin shell grafts versus bone shell grafts for alveolar ridge reconstitution: A novel technique with preliminary results of a prospective clinical study. Int J Periodontics Restorative Dent. 2019;39(6).

79. Um I-W, Kim Y-K, Mitsugi M. Demineralized dentin matrix scaffolds for alveolar bone engineering. J Indian Prosthodont Soc. 2017;17(2):120-7.

80. Umebayashi M, Ohba S, Kurogi T, Noda S, Asahina I. Full Regeneration of Maxillary Alveolar Bone Using Autogenous Partially Demineralized Dentin Matrix and Particulate Cancellous Bone and Marrow for Implant-Supported Full Arch Rehabilitation. J Oral Implantol. 1 Apr 2020;46(2):122-7.

81. Pang K-M, Um I-W, Kim Y-K, Woo J-M, Kim S-M, Lee J-H. Autogenous demineralized dentin matrix from extracted tooth for the augmentation of alveolar bone defect: a prospective randomized clinical trial in comparison with anorganic bovine bone. Clin Oral Implants Res. Jul 2017;28(7):809-15.

82. Minamizato T, Koga T, I T, Nakatani Y, Umebayashi M, Sumita Y, et al. Clinical application of autogenous partially demineralized dentin matrix prepared immediately after extraction for alveolar bone regeneration in implant dentistry: a pilot study. Int J Oral Maxillofac Surg. Jan 2018;47(1):125-32.

83. Korsch M, Peichl M. Retrospective Study: Lateral Ridge Augmentation Using Autogenous Dentin: Tooth-Shell Technique vs. Bone-Shell Technique. Int J Environ Res Public Health. 19 March 2021;18(6):3174.

84. Korsch M. Tooth shell technique: A proof of concept with the use of autogenous dentin block grafts. Aust Dent J. June 2021;66(2):159-68.

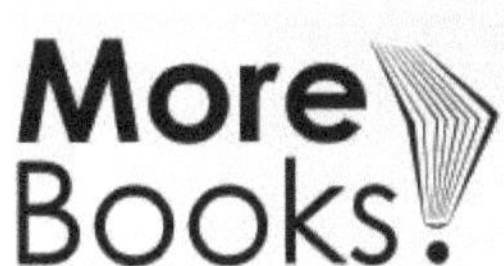

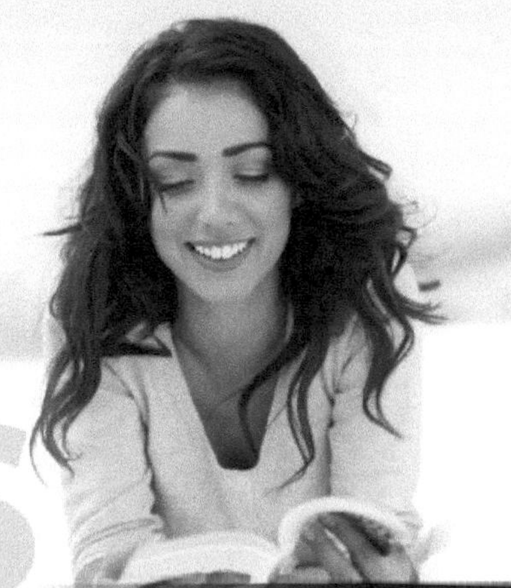

yes **I want** morebooks!

Buy your books fast and straightforward online - at one of world's fastest growing online book stores! Environmentally sound due to Print-on-Demand technologies.

Buy your books online at
www.morebooks.shop

Kaufen Sie Ihre Bücher schnell und unkompliziert online – auf einer der am schnellsten wachsenden Buchhandelsplattformen weltweit! Dank Print-On-Demand umwelt- und ressourcenschonend produziert.

Bücher schneller online kaufen
www.morebooks.shop

info@omniscriptum.com
www.omniscriptum.com

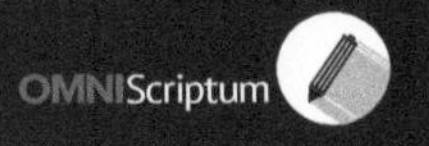

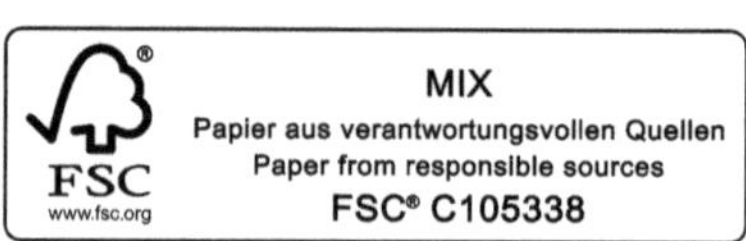

Printed by Books on Demand GmbH, Norderstedt / Germany